IBER5346

TOXICITY ASSESSMENT ALTERNATIVES
METHODS, ISSUES, OPPORTUNITIES

TOXICITY ASSESSMENT
ALTERNATIVES

METHODS, ISSUES, OPPORTUNITIES

Edited by

HARRY SALEM, PHD

*US Army Soldier and Biological
Chemical Command,
Aberdeen Proving Ground, MD*

and

SIDNEY A. KATZ, PHD

Rutgers University, Camden, NJ

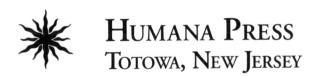

HUMANA PRESS
TOTOWA, NEW JERSEY

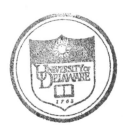

RA
1199
.T66
1999

For additional copies, pricing for bulk purchases, and/or information about other Humana titles, contact Humana at the above address or at any of the following numbers: Tel.: 973-256-1699; Fax: 973-256-8341; E-mail: humana@humanapr.com; Website: http://humanapress.com

Printed in the United States of America. 10 9 8 7 6 5 4 3 2 1

Library of Congress Cataloging in Publication Data

Main entry under title:

Toxicity Assessment Alternatives : methods, issues, opportunities / edited by Harry Salem and Sidney A. Katz
    p.   cm.
    Includes index.
    ISBN 0-89603-787-8 (alk. paper)
    1. Toxicity testing—In vivo—Methodology. 2. Toxicity testing—In vitro—Methodology.   I. Salem, Harry, 1929–   . II. Katz, Sidney A.
    [DNLM: 1. Animal Testing Alternatives. W 20.55A5 T755 1999]
    RA1199.T684   1999
    615.9'07—dc21
    DNLM/DLC
    for Library of Congress   99-21437
                                                               CIP

PREFACE

Toxicity Assessment Alternatives: Methods, Issues, Opportunities contains a broad array of critical surveys, contributed by active and respected investigators, describing their research and offering updates on toxicity assessment alternatives, directions determined by current and future grant programs, opportunities for mechanistically based test methods to detect endocrine disruptor activity, the use of alternatives in the Department of Defense hazard assessment initiatives, and the issues and opportunities for validation and regulatory acceptance.

Several of these advances make use of transgenic models that reduce the time and cost of carcinogenicity testing. Others use tissue cultures for the assessment of endocrine disrupting chemicals. Cultures of human epidermal keratinocytes are applicable as models for sulfur mustard lesions, and in vitro protein denaturation is used as a chemical test for assessing the ocular and dermal irritation potential of cosmetic products. Molecular modeling is applied to explaining chemical toxicity.

Commercially developed assay systems have undergone extensive evaluation by their manufacturers. Some of these await external validation, and others await acceptance by North American and European regulatory agencies.

Toxicity Assessment Alternatives: Methods, Issues, Opportunities provides information from members of the scientific and regulatory communities on what has been achieved and what has been accepted in alternatives to animal testing.

Harry Salem, PhD
Sidney A. Katz, PhD

CONTENTS

CONTRIBUTORS

MICHAEL ASCHNER, PHD, *Department of Physiology and Pharmacology, Bowman Gray School of Medicine of Wake Forest University, Winston-Salem, NC*

MARTIN BELIVEAU, BSC, *Groupe de Recherche en Toxicologic Humaine (TOXHUM), Universite de Montreal, Montreal, PQ, Canada*

BETTY J. BENTON, BS, *US Army Medical Research Institute of Chemical Defense, Aberdeen Proving Ground, MD*

K. RAMACHANDRA BHAT, PHD, *Department of Chemistry, Lincoln University, Lincoln, PA*

JAMES A. BLANK, PHD, *Medical Research and Evaluation Facility, Battelle Memorial Institute, Columbus, OH*

CLARENCE A. BROOMFIELD, PHD, *Biochemical Pharmacology Division, US Army Medical Institute of Chemical Defense, Aberdeen Proving Ground, MD*

C. J. CAO, MD, PHD, *Department of Pharmacology and Experimental Therapeutics, University of Maryland School of Medicine, Baltimore, MD*

HO CHUNG, PHD, *Division of Therapeutics, Department of Pharmacology, Walter Reed Army Institute of Research, Washington, DC; Department of Pharmaceutical Sciences, University of Maryland, Baltimore, MD*

OFFIE E. CLARK, BS, *US Army Medical Research Institute of Chemical Defense, Aberdeen Proving Ground, MD*

PATRICIA D. CONFER, BS, *GEO-Centers Inc., Newton, MA*

FRED M. COWAN, BS, *Biochemical Pharmacology Division, US Army Medical Institute of Chemical Defense, Aberdeen Proving Ground, MD*

RICHARD DICKERSON, PHD, DABT, *Department of Pharmacology, The Institute of Environmental and Human Health, Texas Tech University/Texas Tech Medical Center, Lubbock, TX*

A. T. ELDEFRAWI, PHD, *Department of Pharmacology and Experimental Therapeutics, University of Maryland School of Medicine, Baltimore, MD*

M. E. ELDEFRAWI, PHD, *Department of Pharmacology and Experimental Therapeutics, University of Maryland School of Medicine, Baltimore, MD*

CLARK L. GROSS, MS, *US Army Medical Research Institute of Chemical Defense, Aberdeen Proving Ground, MD*

TRACEY A. HAMILTON, *Veterinary Medicine Division, US Army Medical Research Institute of Chemical Defense, Aberdeen Proving Ground, MD*

JOY L. HARRIS, *Medical Research and Evaluation Facility, Battelle Memorial Institute, Columbus, OH*

KIKI B. HELLMAN, PHD, *Center for Devices and Radiological Health, US Food and Drug Administration, Rockville, MD*

SPIROS P. KATSIFIS, PHD, *Department of Biology, University of Bridgeport, Bridgeport, CT*

JONATHAN W. KAUFMAN, PHD, *Human Performance Technology Branch, Naval Air Warfare Center Aircraft Division, Patuxent River, MD*

SUSAN A. KELLY, BS, *Drug Assessment Division, US Army Medical Research Institute of Chemical Defense, Aberdeen Proving Ground, MD*

RONALD KENDALL, SR., PHD, *Department of Pharmacology, The Institute of Environmental and Human Health, Texas Tech University/Texas Tech Medical Center, Lubbock, TX*

PATRICK L. KINNEY, PHD, *School of Public Health, Division of Environmental Sciences, Columbia University, New York, New York*

STEPHEN D. KIRBY, BS, *Biochemical Pharmacology Branch, US Army Medical Research Institute of Chemical Defense, Aberdeen Proving Ground, MD*

KANNAN KRISHNAN, PHD, *Groupe de Recherche en Toxicologic Humaine (TOXHUM), Universite de Montreal, Montreal, P.Q. Canada*

JOHN C. LIPSCOMB, PHD, *National Center for Environmental Assessment, US Environmental Protection Agency, Cinncinnati, OH*

JANNA S. MADREN-WHALLEY, *Biochemical Pharmacology Branch, US Army Medical Research Institute of Chemical Defense, Aberdeen Proving Ground, MD*

MARGARET E. MARTENS, PHD, *US Army Medical Research Institute of Chemical Defense, Aberdeen Proving Ground, MD*

HENRY L. MEIER, PHD, *Drug Assessment Division, US Army Medical Research Institute of Chemical Defense, Aberdeen Proving Ground, MD*

D. E. MENKING, MS, *Research and Technology Directorate, US Army Edgewood Chemical and Biological Center (USAECBC), Aberdeen Proving Ground, MD*

RONALD G. MENTON, PHD, *Medical Research and Evaluation Facility, Battelle Memorial Institute, Columbus, OH*

CHARLES B. MILLARD, PHD, *US Army Medical Research Institute of Chemical Defense, Aberdeen Proving Ground, MD*

R. J. MIODUSZEWSKI, PHD, *Research and Technology Directorate, US Army Edgewood Chemical and Biological Center (USAECBC), Aberdeen Proving Ground, MD*

DAVID MOIR, PHD, *Department of Systemic Toxicology and Pharmacokinetics, Bureau of Chemical Hazards, Health Canada, Ottawa, Canada*

JANET MOSER, DVM, PHD, *Drug Assessment Division, US Army Medical Research Institute of Chemical Defense, Aberdeen Proving Ground, MD*

PATRICK POULIN, PHD, *Groupe de Recherche en Toxicologic Humaine (TOXHUM), Universite de Montreal, Montreal, P.Q. Canada*

RADHARAMAN RAY, PHD, *US Army Medical Research Institute of Chemical Defense, Aberdeen Proving Ground, MD*

EDITH R. SCHWARTZ , PHD, *Biomed Consultants, Washington, DC*

WILLIAM J. SMITH, PHD, *Biochemical Pharmacology Division, US Army Medical Institute of Chemical Defense, Aberdeen Proving Ground, MD*

REBEKAH A. STARNER, BS, *Medical Research and Evaluation Facility, Battelle Memorial Institute, Columbus, OH*

MARTIN L. STEPHENS, PHD, *Division of Animal Research Issues, The Humane Society of the United States, Washington, DC*

SANJEEV THOHAN, PHD, *Department of Metabolic Chemistry, Covance Laboratories, Madison, WI*

J. J. VALDES, PHD, *Research and Technology Directorate, US Army Edgewood Chemical and Biological Center (USAECBC), Aberdeen Proving Ground, MD*

ROBERT J. WERRLEIN, PHD, *Biochemical Pharmacology Branch, US Army Medical Research Institute of Chemical Defense, Aberdeen Proving Ground, MD*

R. B. WOROBEC, PHD, *Library of Congress, Washington, DC*

ELAINE YOUNG, PHD, *Department of Research, Juvenile Diabetes Foundation International, Washington, DC*

JEFFREY J. YOURICK, PHD, *US Army Medical Research Institute of Chemical Defense, Aberdeen Proving Ground, MD*

ERROL ZEIGER, PHD, JD, *Environmental Toxicology Program, National Institute of Environmental Health Sciences, Research Triangle Park, NC*

I RECENT DEVELOPMENTS ON ALTERNATIVES

1

Tissue Engineering

*An Important Technology
for Assessment of Toxicity*

Edith R. Schwartz, PhD

CONTENTS

INTRODUCTION

The Advanced Technology Program (ATP) at the National Institute of Standards and Technology (NIST) supports, on a cost-shared basis, high-risk technology projects that are likely to have broad-based economic benefits for the US. Project proposals in any area of technology, submitted by a single company or as a joint venture from two or more companies, are judged on a competitive basis both on scientific/technical and economic/business merits. A number of start-up companies dedicated to the development of tissue engineered products have received ATP awards since the program's inception in 1990.

Adverse publicity associated with the use of animals for toxicity testing of cosmetic products first stimulated the search for "in vitro" systems that could serve similar functions. This need, coupled with the emergence of tissue engineering as a recognized discipline, has resulted in research and development dedicated to producing tissue-engineered products to serve as "in vitro" alternatives. Scientists from many disciplines, including molecular and cellular biology, biotechnology and

From: *Toxicity Assessment Alternatives: Methods, Issues, Opportunities*
Edited by: H. Salem and S. A. Katz © Humana Press Inc., Totowa, NJ

3

biochemistry, material science and biomedical engineering, as well as physicians and surgeons have played major roles in discoveries that serve as the bases for the design of these products.

TISSUE ENGINEERING

Tissue engineering integrates discoveries about cells and biomaterials to produce innovative three-dimensional (3-D) composites that have structure/function properties that can be used either to correct or replace defective tissues/organs "in vivo," or to measure the effects of external influences on such structures "in vitro." The material components may be processed from naturally derived or synthetic substances, or combinations of these. The cellular components may be of human or animal origin.

Biomaterials

Native, chemically modified, derivatized and/or polymeric forms of compounds listed in Table 1 are being incorporated into tissue-engineered products either as scaffolding, coating, or encapsulating materials. Certain molecular entities of these materials already have received FDA approval for other uses, such as vehicles for drug delivery or as surgical tools. Among unique features of these compounds is the ability to modify the basic structures in multiple ways while retaining comparable biocompatibility. Furthermore, these materials can be chemically and physically altered to achieve changing rates of bioresorption as well as variations in physical parameters, such as tensile strength, elastic modulus, and pore size. Cell-binding properties can be promoted by inclusion of adhesion molecules. For some situations, it appears that composites of two or more of these materials may be preferred. This is particularly relevant if pH or other microenvironmental factors need to be controlled during the resorption period. Although the successful weaving together of appropriate biomaterials and cells into commercially viable tissue-engineered products is being actively pursued in numerous laboratories, it will be several years before many of these products are approved and become readily available in the marketplace.

Cells

Table 2 lists some of the cell types presently in test systems of tissue-engineered products for diagnostic and therapeutic use. Each cell type has unique features that are captured in the devices in development. Results from initial clinical trials indicate that injection of normal myoblasts, proliferated in vitro, into diseased muscles of individuals with muscular dystrophy produces amelioration of the disease in some patients *(1)*. In a different disease area, clinical trials have demonstrated

Table 1
Biomaterials Used in Tissue-Engineered Products

Collagen	Proteoglycans
Glycosaminoglycans	Laminin
Polylactic acid	Hydroxyapatite
Polyglycolic acid	Hyaluronic acid
Alginate derivatives	Polycaprolactone
Tyrosine-derived polycarbonates	

Table 2
Cell Types Used
in Tissue-Engineered Products

Muscle	Dermal
Fibroblasts	Chondrocytes
Hepatocytes	β Islet
Bone	Keratinocytes
Stem	

that when attached to the circulatory system of a patient with chronic liver disease, an extracorporeal device containing normal hepatocytes in a biocompatible matrix was able to remove the toxic elements from the patient's blood *(2)*. Most recently, research interests have focused on multipotential stem cells. Several investigators have shown that differentiation of these cells can be regulated in numerous ways, including variations in physical forces, addition of growth factors, and by changing the composition of the extracellular matrix in which these cells are cultivated *(3)*. It has been proposed that storage of primitive cells isolated from the umbilical cord of newborns may become a universal source of cells for tissue-engineered products in the future.

Regulatory Approval

The first tissue-regenerative product to receive FDA approval was a dermal regeneration template for skin repair in burn patients, which had been developed by Integra LifeSciences Inc., a biotechnology company in Plainsboro, NJ. The invention was based on technology licensed from M.I.T. and the Massachusetts General Hospital. The company is expanding its tissue-engineering efforts and, with the help of an ATP award, now is developing new technologies for use in bone repair. This work, performed in collaboration with the Department of Chemistry at Rutgers University and The Department of Bioengineering at The Hospital for Joint Diseases in New York City, aims to exploit the properties of the newly synthesized tyrosine polycarbonates for devices that will have superior properties in orthopedic applications.

Another dermal-related product that is on the market is an "in vitro" device that is used to evaluate the effects of cosmetics, household agents and drugs on skin. Skin2™, commercialized by Advanced Tissue Sciences, Inc., San Diego, CA is an "in vitro" laboratory testing kit consisting of a three-dimensional dermal, full-thickness, or barrier function model skin substrate that is used for testing cytotoxicity, irritancy, percutaneous absorption, wound healing, and phototoxicity *(4)*. Although used principally for "in vitro" testing of new ingredients for potential skin and eye irritation by cosmetic, pharmaceutical, and household products companies, the US Department of Transportation recently approved the product for corrosivity testing. Despite these successes, many scientific, technical, and manufacturing challenges remain to be overcome before an additional number of new, effective, reproducible, and affordable tissue-engineered products appear either on the diagnostic or therapeutic markets.

Manufacturing

The identification, isolation, proliferation, maintenance, and genetic alteration of cells for use in tissue-engineered products are being pursued actively in many laboratories. Among the hurdles facing developers of these products are the needs to

1. Design improved fermentation-type bioreactors for large-scale culturing of human and/or animal cells.
2. Find better sterilization procedures that will not alter cell properties.
3. Develop more efficient methods to freeze and store cells in order to minimize the loss of viability during these processes.

As noted, the proper combination of cells and biomaterials eventually will serve as "in vitro" test systems to examine the safety of newly developed cosmetic, household, and pharmaceutical ingredients as well as of industrial products given off into the environment. Furthermore, the effects of infectious agents, including viruses, on different cell types may be monitored in these systems. To maximize the social and economic benefits, these products must be fabricated to have a long shelf life and packaged in a cost-effective way so that they may be easily transported and made available on a global basis. This requires packaging in heat-stable containers that if necessary, can withstand freezing and thawing. Manufacturing know-how from other industries is being applied to reduce the cost and improve the quality of tissue-engineered products. For example, Tissue Engineering Inc. of Boston, MA, a recipient of an early ATP award, has modified textile knitting equipment to produce novel forms of biomaterials that have the necessary surface composition and the needed ratios of surface areas and porosity for maximum cell interaction.

THE ROLE OF ATP

Although the greatest use of tissue-engineered products in the future will be to replace structurally or physiologically deficient or diseased tissues and/or organs in humans, the "in vitro" market is an important auxiliary area that will serve both as a test system for the newly developed devices as well as a revenue stream for the companies involved in the research, development, and marketing of these products.

At this time, tissue-engineered products are being developed principally by small "start-up" companies that have in-licensed the intellectual property on which the proposed technology development is based. Recently organized regional tissue-engineering initiatives in several communities, including Pittsburgh, Houston, San Francisco, and Boston, have spawned several such companies. Although initial feasibility studies have been positive, technical challenges and risks remain. As a result of ATP funding of projects in tissue engineering, companies have been able to attract additional investments, shorten the R&D cycle of their potential products, engage in public offerings, and form collaborations and strategic alliances.

For example, two companies have received ATP support to help develop tissue-engineered products to treat diabetes. These devices, when injected into the patient, would help maintain normal glucose levels. In the US alone, the estimated direct and indirect health care costs associated with diabetes was about $100 billion in 1995. These two projects are similar in that they focus on the development of physiologic biomaterials that circumvent immune rejection, and on improved methods for the isolation, proliferation, and encapsulation of β islet cells. In addition, both companies are devising newer manufacturing technologies to produce these tissue-engineered therapies in mass quantities. Despite the common objectives of these projects, there are significant substantive differences in the methods and materials that are being discovered and developed.

VivoRx Inc., a start-up biotechnology company in Santa Monica, CA, is developing encapsulated β islet cells or organoids that are contained in immunoprotective microcapsules composed of a novel photopolymerizable alginate material. With ATP support, the company has designed and built a prototype device to manufacture microcapsules with reproducible strength, shape, size, and chemical stability. Additionally, ATP support is being used to discover improved methods for cell proliferation and the development of newer alginate derivatives with increased biocompatibility. Initial studies have shown normaliza-

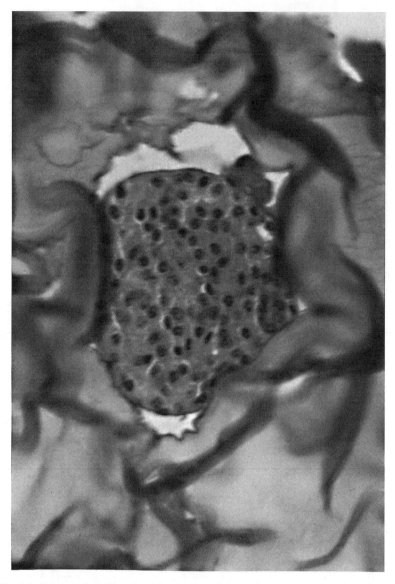

Fig. 1A. Encapsulated bovine islet retrieved from the peritoneal cavity of a dog 6 wk after xenotransplantation **(A,B)** *(5)*.

tion of insulin levels in experimental animals that have been treated with these organoids.

With funding provided by ATP, BioHybrid Technologies Inc., a start-up biotechnology company in Shrewsbury, MA, in collaboration with Synergy Research Corporation of New Hampshire, is developing

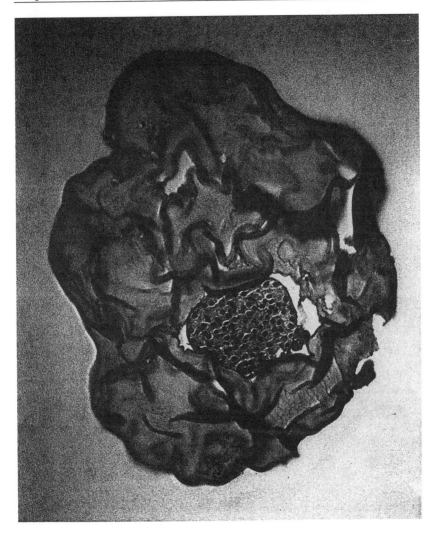

Fig. 1B

microreactors that contain living β islet cells. The microreactors are surrounded by a permaselective membrane that makes them impervious to large molecules, such as IgG, but permits the transport of molecules, such as insulin and glucose. Quality-control procedures have been developed to monitor reproducibility of membrane thickness, transport properties, and mechanical strength of microreactors. Tests conducted in diabetic animals have shown that injection of these microreactors can bring the insulin levels back to normal values and that these devices function for several months. This is shown in Fig. 1, which depicts an

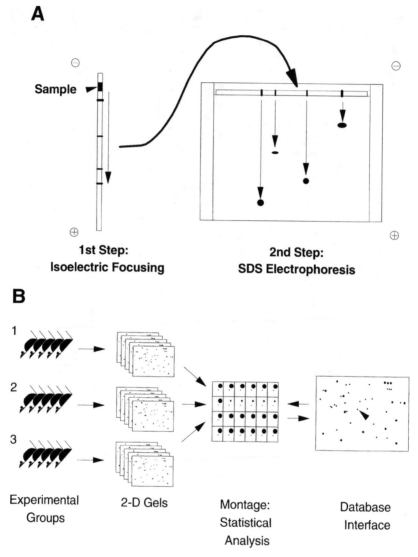

Fig. 2. Principles of operation and analysis of 2-D electrophoresis. **(A)** Fundamental steps of isoelectric focusing in the first direction followed by SDS electrophoresis in the second direction. **(B)** Statistical analysis of high-resolution patterns of multiple samples reflecting identical experimental conditions to identify and characterize a particular spot representing a single protein species (N. G. Anderson, personal communication).

Fig. 3. *(opposite page)* Master 2-D gel pattern of proteins from rat liver. Multiple electrophoretic patterns of liver samples obtained from a large number of animals were analyzed as depicted in Fig. 2. Arrows indicate proteins that have been identified by amino-acid sequencing (N. G. Anderson, personal communication).

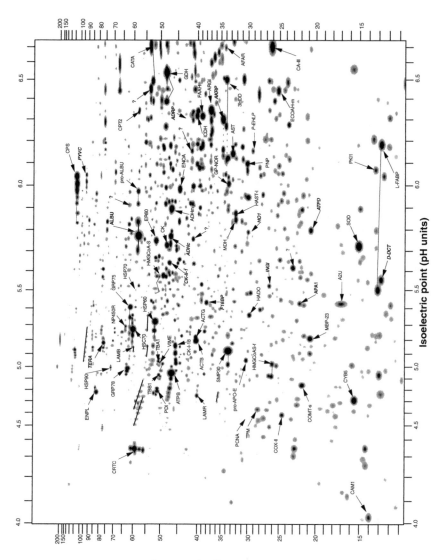

Molecular Weight (kDaltons)

Isoelectric point (pH units)

encapsulated bovine islet retrieved from the peritoneal cavity of a dog 6 wk after xenotransplantation. The company presently is investigating ways to expand the production of these microreactors, since it will need large quantities for use in clinical trials.

Clinical trials and FDA approval for products from either or both of these companies for therapeutic use will take many years. In the interim, however, the scientific principles that serve as the bases for these projects can be used to produce tissue-engineered devices that may be applicable for "in vitro" examination of potential drugs to treat diabetes as well as to learn more about genetic or environmental factors that could be responsible for the onset of the disease. Furthermore, these devices are generic in nature, and their use, therefore, may be expanded to examine other diseases by altering the cell type or the encapsulating material.

A totally different approach to support "in vitro" toxicity testing is being taken by Large Scale Biology Corporation (LSB) of Rockville, MD. With support from ATP, LSB is developing advanced two-dimensional (2-D) electrophoresis systems that incorporate protein index databases, computer analysis of 2-D gels, and newly designed automatic electrophoretic systems. Based on statistical analyses of patterns obtained following the fundamental 2-D system of isoelectric focusing in the first direction and SDS electrophoresis in the second step (Figs. 2A,B) of multiple samples, the company has developed identifying maps of hundreds of proteins. One such map, representing proteins present in rat liver, is shown in Fig. 3. The proteins, visualized on the gels either with Coomassie blue or silver stain, are isolated and then identified by amino acid sequencing. Changes in the source material would be represented by changes in the maps' patterns. For example, as indicated by the arrows in Fig. 4, the concentration of liver HMG-CoA Synthase, an enzyme involved in cholesterol metabolism, responds in a quantitative way to the administration of cholesterol-lowering agents in experimental animals with high levels of cholesterol. It is anticipated that similar results would be found with the use of hepatocytes in a three-dimensional tissue-engineered liver system "in vitro." In time, the expectation is that the databases will be sufficiently comprehensive to permit their use early in the drug development cycle to detect potential toxicity problems or to validate apparent safety and efficacy.

Fig. 4. *(opposite page)* A montage of 2-D electrophoretic patterns of rat liver, showing effects of four cholesterol-altering treatments vs control. All treatment compounds were administered to five male F344 rats in diet at the concentrations shown for 7 d. An arrow indicates the principal spot comprising cytosolic HMG-CoA-synthase. Reproduced with permission *(6)*.

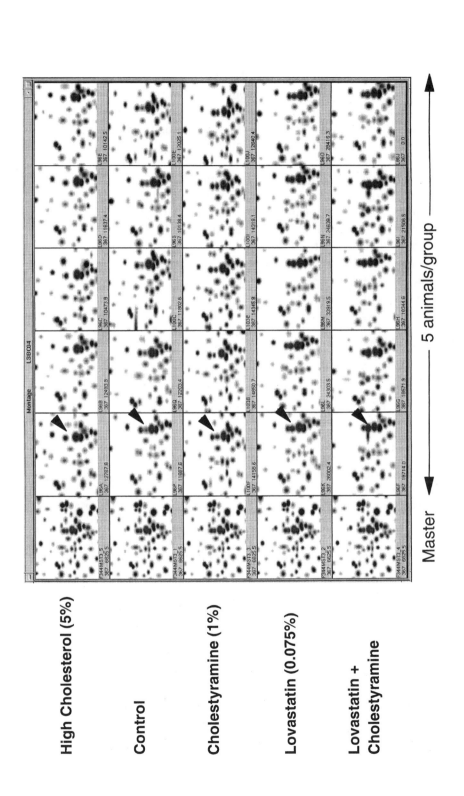

High Cholesterol (5%)

Control

Cholestyramine (1%)

Lovastatin (0.075%)

Lovastatin + Cholestyramine

Master ◀——————— 5 animals/group ———————▶

DISCUSSION

The near completion of the Human Genome Project has provided the information necessary to identify many of the genes, and consequently the proteins, that convey specificity of form and function to cells during human development. These data are extremely valuable in verifying the integrity and stability of tissue-engineered products, since in many ways, their formation parallels such development. Furthermore, recent reports from several laboratories suggest that the physical makeup and the chemical composition of the extracellular matrix have profound effects on cell differentiation, dedifferentiation and transdifferentiation. This would indicate that almost any tissue or organ can be simulated by placing the correct cell type into an appropriate extracellular matrix. In the future, therefore, it is likely that tissue-engineered products will be designed by computers having databases that describe specific interactions between cells and materials in defined chemical and physical environments. In this way, "in vitro" testing of new compounds could become universally available at reasonable costs.

REFERENCES

1. Law PK. *Whole body treatment*. In: Myoblast Transfer: Gene Therapy for Muscular Dystrophy. Law PK, ed., CRC, Austin, 1994; pp. 121–135.
2. Sussman NL, Gislason GT, Conlin CA, Kelly JH. The hepatic extracorporeal liver assist device: Initial clinical experience. Artif Organs 1994;18:390–396.
3. Migliaccio G, Baiocchi M, Hamel N, Eddleman K, Migliaccio AR. Circulating progenitor cells in human ontogenesis: Response to growth factors and regulating potential. J Hematotherapeut 1996;5:161–170.
4. Whalen E, Donnelly TA, Naughton G, Rheins LA. The Development of three-dimensional in vitro human tissue models. Hum Exp Toxicol 1994;12:853–859.
5. Lanza RP, Kuhtreiber WM, Ecker JP, Ecker DM, Marsh JP, Staruck OE, Chick WI. Xenotransplantation of bovine islets into dogs using biodegradable, injectable microreactors. Transplantation Proceedings 1996;28:828 (by permission).
6. Anderson NG, Anderson HL. Twenty years of two-dimensional electrophoresis: past, present and future. Electrophoresis 1996;17:443.

2

Tissue Engineering
Technology Applications and FDA Initiatives

Kiki B. Hellman, PHD

ADVANCES IN TISSUE ENGINEERING

Tissue engineering has emerged over the past 10–15 years as a novel technology that uses the concepts and tools of biotechnology, molecular and cell biology, materials science, and engineering to understand the structure–function relationships in mammalian tissues *(1)*, and to develop biological substitutes for the repair, reconstruction, regeneration, or replacement of tissue function *(2)*. As a source of products and systems, tissue engineering has emerged at the interface between the medical device and biotechnology industries *(3)*.

Biological substitutes generally consist of living cells or tissues and biomaterials. A variety of cells or tissues, either native or genetically manipulated, from human or animal sources can be used. Sources for biomaterials include materials of natural origin or synthetic materials developed for specific chemical or physical properties. Biomaterials are used to:

1. Provide a scaffold or three-dimensional (3-D) architecture for tissue regeneration.
2. Modulate a specific cell function.
3. Provide immunoprotection *(3)*.

From: *Toxicity Assessment Alternatives: Methods, Issues, Opportunities*
Edited by: H. Salem and S. A. Katz © Humana Press Inc., Totowa, NJ

There are many types of products in different stages of development that promise major advances in clinical medicine. They range from wound covering/repair and bone/cartilage repair systems to cardiovascular tissue-engineered devices, drug delivery systems, and encapsulated cells for restoration of tissue and organ function. These products are indicative of the novel therapeutic approaches developed through advances in tissue engineering that combine the delivery of pharmacologically active substances, elements of medical devices, biological products, and surgical interventions *(3)*.

Cultures of structural, secretory, and other cells, tissues, or organs developed for tissue-engineered products can also be utilized as in vitro model systems for evaluating modulation of structure and/or function by toxicological and other agents.

SCIENTIFIC AND REGULATORY ISSUES

Tissue-engineered products will be subject to regulatory evaluation by the national agencies responsible for overseeing the approval for the commercial distribution of medical products before they are admitted to the armamentarium of clinical medicine. Issues of product safety and efficacy as they relate to product manufacture, preclinical evaluation, clinical investigation, and postmarket requirements will be considered in this evaluation.

The FDA Tissue Engineering Working Group was established to address the scientific and regulatory issues of tissue-engineered products. The Working Group has identified certain generic safety and effectiveness issues for consideration by the community in its development of products. Examples range from considerations for cell/tissue sourcing and characterization, testing for adventitious agents, and characterization of biomaterials components and demonstration of biomaterial compatibility to product consistency and stability, appropriate preclinical in vitro and animal models, clinical study design, and end points for clinical safety and efficacy *(2)*.

FDA centers are using different approaches in the evaluation of tissue-engineered products. These include:

1. Research (bioeffects analysis and testing; test method development).
2. Data and information monitoring (databases).
3. Regulatory guidance (generic product-specific and points to consider).
4. Training and education (FDA staff colleges; workshops/conferences).
5. Cooperation with public and private groups.

INTERNATIONAL DIALOGUE AND HARMONIZATION STRATEGY

As tissue-engineered products assume a worldwide marketplace, assurance of consistent regulatory procedures among different countries for the evaluation of these products becomes more important. A common regulatory approach is a critical element for reaping the public health benefits worldwide. To this end, an understanding of the pre- and postmarket regulatory requirements for tissue-engineered products, together with the rationale (paradigm) and approaches used in the regulatory evaluation by the different responsible national agencies, are important in the ultimate development of an international dialogue and a global regulatory perspective for these products.

REFERENCES

1. Hellman KB, Picciolo GL, Fox CF. Prospects for Application of biotechnology-derived biomaterials. J Cell Biochem 1994;56:210–224.
2. Hellman KB. Biomedical applications of tissue engineering technology: regulatory issues. Tissue Eng 1995;1:2:203–210.
3. Galletti PM, Hellman KB, Nerem RM. Tissue engineering: from basic science to products: a preface. Tissue Eng 1995;1:2:147–149.

3

Electrical Resistance Method for Measuring Volume Changes in Astrocytes

Michael Aschner, PhD

CONTENTS

INTRODUCTION
ASTROCYTIC SWELLING
MEASUREMENTS OF ASTROCYTIC VOLUME
    WITH THE ELECTRICAL RESISTANCE MODEL
SUMMARY
ACKNOWLEDGMENT
REFERENCES

INTRODUCTION

The term edema was coined to describe the pathological condition of brain swelling. Associated with brain swelling are cessation of blood supply owing to raised intracranial pressure (ICP) and displacement of central nervous system (CNS) tissue, since the closed confines of the skull and meninges do not accommodate outward expansion of the CNS. Early workers in this field have differentiated between two types of brain swelling. One involved the extracellular accumulation of water and was termed edema (derived from the Greek word Oidema, which means swelling). Its diagnostic feature was that the cut brain "wept fluid." It was differentiated from brain swelling, which was thought to be intracellular swelling, characterized by the dryness of the cut brain. The pioneering work of Klatzo *(1)* resolved many of the ambiguities

From: *Toxicity Assessment Alternatives: Methods, Issues, Opportunities*
Edited by: H. Salem and S. A. Katz © Humana Press Inc., Totowa, NJ

regarding brain edema and its etiologies. Studying myelin swelling on triethyltin (TET) exposure, Klatzo redefined brain edema as a generic term to describe excessive accumulation of fluid within the brain. He distinguished, however, between two types of brain edema: (1) vasogenic edema, where injury to the vessel wall and compromised function of the blood–brain barrier lead to escape of water and plasma exudates into the brain parenchyma, and (2) cytotoxic edema in which toxic compounds directly affect the cellular elements, leading to intracellular swelling in the absence of changes in the restrictive properties of the blood–brain barrier. Nevertheless, Klatzo pointed out that in vivo both types of CNS swelling are usually likely to coexist.

Since cytotoxic edema is the most common observed component of brain swelling, this chapter will be restricted to this type of swelling, outlining its most general aspects. For a recent review on vasogenic edema, the reader is referred to a review by Kimelberg et al. *(2)*. Furthermore, because astrocytes are commonly swollen in brain trauma of various etiologies, this chapter will mainly focus on this cell type, discussing swelling mechanisms in these cells in some detail. Finally, a newly developed electrical resistance method for measuring volume changes in astrocytes and its potential to serve as a screening method for neurotoxicity will be described, emphasizing mechanisms associated with the inhibition of astrocyte volume regulation on exposure to the organic metal, methylmercury (MeHg).

ASTROCYTIC SWELLING

Astrocytic Swelling: Mechanisms

Astrocytes occupy approx 20% of the cell volume of the gray matter, and their processes are found around synapses and in close apposition to the nodes of Ranvier, axon tracts, and the capillaries. Functions ascribed to astrocytes include the elaboration and secretion of neurotrophic factors, control of the interstitial pH, concentrative uptake and metabolism of neurotransmitters, modulation of neuronal signals, immune modulation, and tissue repair, just to name a few. Since review of astrocytic functions is beyond the scope of this chapter, the reader is referred to a number of comprehensive reviews on this topic *(3–9)*. Astrocytes are commonly swollen in brain trauma, and astrocytic swelling is an important early event, predisposing the brain to further damage because of the impairment of important homeostatic, protective astrocytic functions. Therefore, when astrocytic functions are disarmed, the consequences to the CNS as a whole may be disastrous.

The mechanisms of astrocytic swelling, although still ill-defined, have yielded to in vitro analysis owing to the availability of pure primary astrocyte cultures. It appears, at least in its exaggerated form, that astrocytic swelling is deleterious or a true pathology. Persistent astrocytic swelling can be viewed as a pathological extension of more limited and controlled volume changes that are otherwise part of the normal homeostatic function of astrocytes. Astroglial swelling, such as in experimental ischemia, has been extensively studied. It prominently involves swelling of the cell body as well as the astrocytic foot processes around both neurons and capillaries $(10,11)$. By means of electron microscopy, such swelling is recognized as a pale and a watery cytoplasm, distinct from the hypertrophy in reactive astrogliosis where the cell cytoplasm is packed with glial fibrillary acidic protein- (GFAP) positive intermediate filaments.

Astrocytic swelling is a complex phenomenon, with at least four different contributing mechanisms, which may operate alone or in tandem. The four most common mechanisms are schematically depicted in Fig. 1. The first swelling mechanism, termed acid-base or pH-driven, invokes the simultaneous operation of Cl^-/HCO_3^- and Na^+/H^+ exchange transport systems, with H^+ and HCO_3^- cycling from the intra- to extracellular spaces via membrane-permeant CO_2 $(12,13)$. It has also been demonstrated that glutamate (glutamate-driven swelling; Fig. 1) can lead to volumetric enlargement of astrocytes when injected directly into the CNS (14). Glutamate is likely to operate by increasing production of the metabolic products CO_2 and H^+, thus leading to swelling by similar processes to those described above. In addition, astrocytes transport glutamate intracellularly by an Na^+-dependent mechanism, which is also dependent on K^+ efflux (15). This transport (glutamate-driven; Fig. 1) has a likely stoichiometry of one glutamate and three Na^+ transported inwardly, and one K^+ transported outwardly to offset the negative charge of glutamate. Such net uptake of Na^+ and glutamate can lead to swelling. Thus, swelling could be owing to direct receptor activation leading to Na^+ entry. Cl^- or HCO_3^- could presumably enter through anion channels, which may also open under these conditions. Increased $[K^+]_o$ (>20 mM), commonly seen in stroke and head injury, is also likely to cause astrocytic swelling by uptake of KCl owing to Donnan forces (16) (Fig. 1). K^+ uptake occurs via K^+ channels, of which there are several types in astrocytes (19); Cl^- uptake occurs largely via Cl^- channels. The Cl^- channels in astrocytes are usually not open at the resting membrane potential, but the large conductance anion channel and smaller conductance Cl^- channels are voltage-sensitive and are activated by swelling $(17,18)$. Finally, volumetric enlargement of astro-

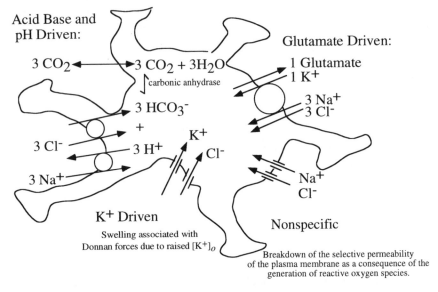

Fig. 1. Mechanisms associated with astrocytic swelling. Acid-base and pH driven: CO_2 readily diffuses through the cell membrane and reacts with intracellular H_2O to form H_2CO_3 in the presence of the zinc-requiring enzyme, carbonic anhydrase (CA). H_2CO_3 readily dissociates in the cell to form H^+ and HCO_3^-. Under normal conditions, pH homeostasis is maintained mainly by the concurrent activity of the Cl^-/HCO_3^- and Na^+/H^+ antiporters. Under conditions of extracellular acidity, the intracellular acidity increases, H^+ is exchanged for Na^+, HCO_3^- is exchanged for Cl^-, and the intracellular concentration of Na^+ and Cl^- rises with the rising H^+ concentration. The extruded H^+ returns to the extracellular space and reacts with HCO_3^- to form more CO_2, which diffuses through the cell membrane. During pathological astrocytic swelling, carbon dioxide clearance decreases and the cell takes on osmotically obligated H_2O and fails to pump out the excess Na^+ and Cl^-, since transporters and Na^+/K^+ ATPase function are compromised. Glutamate-driven: Uptake of excess glutamate with 3 Na^+ (probably 3 Na^+ in and 1 K^+ out). K^+-Driven: Uptake of KCl owing to increased $[K^+]_o$ as a consequence of neuronal activity or energy failure. Nonspecific: Free radicals damage membranes, consequently altering the membrane permeability to ions, and allowing the influx of sodium, chloride, and water. Additional information is provided in the text.

cytes can also result from nonspecific breakdown of the selective permeability of the plasma membrane (nonspecific; Fig. 1), as a consequence of the generation of reactive oxygen species (ROS). ROS are implicated in the etiology of a number of pathologies, both because of the observed generation of free radicals *(19,20)*, and the fact that antioxidants are effective in attenuating the deleterious effects seen in animal models of ischemia and trauma *(21)*.

Astrocytic Swelling: Consequences

Astrocytes in vitro release a number of excitatory amino acids (EAAs) and K^+ in response to a variety of stimuli *(22)*, including elevated $[K^+]_o$ *(23,24)*, mechanical stretching and receptor activation *(25)*, and reduced osmolarity *(26)*. On exposure to hypotonic medium, astrocytes swell and then reshrink towards their normal size, a process referred to as regulatory volume decrease or RVD *(27,28)*. A common mechanism of RVD involves activation of conductive K^+ and Cl^- channels, allowing for the escape of KCl and osmotically obligated water. It had been recently suggested that volume changes control the activity of various channels (such as the ClC-2 channel) by a "ball-and-chain" mechanism. On swelling, the ball, which normally blocks the channel pore, is dislodged, activating the channel *(29)* and allowing for the passive diffusion of ions. Astrocytic exposure to reduced osmolarity is also associated with the release of D-aspartate, L-glutamate, and taurine *(23,25,28,30)*. Whereas taurine plays an important role as an osmolyte *(28,30)*, both aspartate and glutamate do not appear to contribute substantially to cell volume regulation *(24,31,32)*.

Reports on hypotonic-induced ion and amino acid release invoke phosphatidylinositol hydrolysis and elevated $[Ca^{2+}]_i$ as regulatory mechanisms of RVD *(33–35)*. cAMP, calmodulin, eicosanoids, protein kinases, leukotrienes, and the microfilament network have also been postulated to play a role in RVD *(35)*. O'Connor and Kimelberg *(24)* have reported that removal of external calcium can inhibit RVD, at least over the initial 8–10 min, and Bender et al. *(36)* have reported that calmodulin inhibitors inhibit RVD in astrocytes. Studies from our laboratory *(31)*, corroborate a regulatory role for calcium in RVD. Nimodipine, a specific blocker of the L-type calcium channel, significantly inhibited volume regulation. When intracellular calcium was quenched, using 1, 2-*bis*-(2-aminophenoxy)-ethane-N, N, N', N'-tetraacetic acid (tetra[acetoxymethyl] ester) (BAPTA-AM), RVD was inhibited to an even greater extent. Likewise, trifluoperazine, a calmodulin inhibitor, also inhibited RVD. In all of these cases, $[^3H]$-D-aspartate release was significantly increased compared to hypotonic-induced release. In contrast, ^{86}Rb (a marker for K^+) efflux was significantly decreased by these agents. The observation that astrocytes exposed to calcium-free media or nimodipine on hypotonic-induced swelling exhibited some RVD, although at a slower rate than controls, points to a role for intracellular calcium mobilization in RVD *(31)*.

In vivo, significant hyposmolality is almost always owing to lowered plasma Na^+ concentration, i.e., hyponatremia. Hyponatremia is a very common clinical problem occurring in the hospitalized elderly or infants, chronic alcoholics, and in people with kidney disease *(37)*. In response to hypernatremia, the brain either gains electrolytes or non-electrolytes, or synthesizes some of the latter, in order to prevent cell shrinkage. Conversely, it loses electrolytes and nonelectrolytes in hyponatremia. These patterns are very similar to the loss of KCl, glutamate, and taurine, which occur in vitro when cultured astrocytes are swollen in hypotonic medium *(23,31)* or the gain in nonelectrolytes by cultured glia exposed to hyperosmotic solutions *(38)*. Although we do not propose that astrocytes in vivo, other than in hyponatremia or in some form of neonatal renal disease, swell because of decreased extracellular osmolality, we assume as a working hypothesis that the swelling of the astrocytes *in situ*, by whatever mechanism, activates the same ion or amino acid transport processes activated by hypotonic-media-induced swelling in vitro.

This leads to the hypothesis that when astrocytes swell in vivo, they release excitotoxic compounds, such as L-glutamate, which then cause neuronal injury owing to excessive activation of glutamate receptors, leading to cell swelling and influx of Ca^{2+}, according to the excitotoxicity concept *(22)*. This hypothesis is supported by the protective effects of L-644,711 seen in an animal model of closed head injury with hypoxia, where it has been shown to inhibit astrocytic swelling and caused improvements in outcome *(39)*. In vitro, L-644,711 also inhibits swelling-activated release of [^{3}H] L-glutamate from swollen astrocytes *(23)*.

MEASUREMENTS OF ASTROCYTIC VOLUME WITH THE ELECTRICAL RESISTANCE MODEL

Methodology

Astrocytic volumetric changes are measured in our laboratory by a modified dynamic method that is based on the measurement of electrical resistance *(40)*. This, as well as other approaches to volume measurement, highlighting their advantages and disadvantages were previously reviewed *(41)*. Astrocytes are grown on cover slips and placed in a perfusion chamber containing a channel (channel height is 100 μm) bridged between two silver wire electrodes (approx 5 cm in length). Leads from the gold electrodes are made of insulated copper wire, soldered to the silver with pure indium, and the connections are covered with wax (a molten solution of 50% Apiezon M grease and 50% paraffin wax). The gold electrodes are connected through a large resistor (1 MΩ) to a lock-in amplifier (5301, EG & G Princeton Applied Research, Princeton, NJ) that supplies a 500-Hz, 5-V signal to the system. The lock-in amplifier is used, because it is able to resolve small voltage changes with high noise rejection. At the 500 Hz frequency, the cell membranes are insulating, and current will travel over and not through the cell monolayer. Apart from the solution in the channel, the two chambers are insulated from each other.

In a typical experiment, the control bathing medium for all experiments consists of the following: 22 mM NaCl, 3.3 mM KCl, 0.4 mM MgSO$_4$, 1.3 mM CaCl$_2$, 1.2 mM KH$_2$PO$_4$, 10 mM D-(+)-glucose, 25 mM N-2-hydroxyethylpiperazine N'-2-ethanesulfonic acid (HEPES) and 200 mM mannitol. HEPES-buffered solutions are maintained at pH 7.4 by addition of 1 N NaOH. The osmolality of the solutions is approx 300 mosm as measured by a freezing point osmometer (Advanced Instruments, Inc., Needham Heights, MA). Hyposmotic solutions are made by removing the mannitol. The replacement of part of the NaCl with mannitol in isosmotic solutions has the important feature of maintaining the same electrolyte concentration in the respective iso- and hyposmotic solutions, assuring identical conductivity properties. However, a small correction has to be made for the small decrease in solution conductance owing to mannitol, which is corrected for by adding a small amount of water. It is clearly critical to balance all the experimental solutions to the same resistivity so that the resistance (and voltage) differences measured when the solutions are changed can be accounted for solely because of changes in cell volume. Prior to experimentation, the resistivities of the solutions are checked by measuring the solutions over a blank cover slip in the perfusion chamber. The resistivities of paired isosmotic and hyposmotic solutions (or any other experimental solution) are then balanced to within 0.5% by adding small amounts of water to the hypotonic buffer.

The premise of the electrical resistance measurement is simple. As cells swell, their volume increases such that the volume of the solution within the channel available for current flow decreases proportionally, resulting in an increase in measured resistance in the channel above the cells. Since $V = IR$ (where V is voltage, I is current, and R is resistance), and I is constant (500 Hz), changes in V are directly proportional to changes in R. Since the resistance of the chamber itself is <0.02 MΩ, this arrangement essentially provides the system with a constant current source (40). The height of the astrocytic cell monolayer can also be calculated from the resistance measurement of the channel. The cover slip may be removed at the end of each experiment, a blank cover slip can be reintroduced into the chamber, and the difference between the channel resistance under those two experimental conditions equates to the difference in height owing to the cell monolayer. The resting height of the astrocytic monolayer is normally about 5 μM, as determined by this method. The chamber is designed to have a height of approx 100 μm above the cells. Since the method measures the percentage change in voltage (and resistance), a 1% change in the measurement translates to approx 1 μm change in the average cell height of the monolayer. A recorded increase in the voltage (and thus resistance) means that the volume through the channel above the cells available for current flow has decreased by the same amount as the volume of the monolayer cell height has increased.

Each experiment is initiated by placing a #1 cover slip (2.5 × 1.0 cm) on which a confluent monolayer of astrocytes is growing in the channel and continuously perfusing it with isotonic solution at room temperature. If desired, the chamber may be placed in an incubator, and experiments can be conducted at 37°C. The flow through the chamber is driven by hydrostatic pressure (owing to height difference between the solutions and chamber). A pump may also be utilized.

Effects of Mercurials on Astrocytic Volume

MeHg is a particular threat to the CNS in humans *(42,43)*. The case for significant toxicity of MeHg CNS is strongly supported by both in vivo and in vitro studies. That astrocytes play a pivotal role in the etiology of MeHg-induced neurotoxicity is consistent with the following evidence:

1. In vivo, MeHg preferentially accumulates in astrocytes, both in humans and nonhuman primates *(44–46)*.
2. In vitro, MeHg inhibits glutamate and K^+ uptake in astrocytes *(47,48)*. Other transport systems examined are two- to fivefold less sensitive than glutamate to inhibition by MeHg *(49,50)*.
3. In the absence of extracellular glutamate, cultured neurons are unaffected by acute exposure to mercury (Hg) *(51)*.
4. Exposure of astrocytes to MeHg is associated with astrocytic swelling both in vivo *(44–46)* and in vitro, inhibition of RVD, and increased release of endogenous excitatory amino acids (EAAs), such as glutamate and aspartate *(48)*.

The overall aim of our laboratory continues to be to elucidate the mechanisms of MeHg neurotoxicity, postulating that a direct toxic effect of MeHg on astrocytes leads to astrocytic swelling and release of EAAs, which in turn results in neuronal impairment, injury, and death by an excitotoxic mechanism.

Figure 2 depicts the effect of 10 μM MeHg on astrocytic RVD employing the electrical resistance measurement. MeHg significantly inhibits RVD in Na^+-containing hypotonic buffer. The figure shows the calculated change in height of the monolayer above the resting height of the monolayer (5 μm) after exposure to hypotonic buffer. Hypotonically swollen cells achieve maximal height (volume) within 3–5 min after introduction to hypotonic buffer (t = 18–20 min; maximal volume, MV) (~3 μm increase in average cell height), and thereafter begin to volume regulate. Within 30 min of exposure to hypotonicity, untreated cells had volume regulated to within 0.5 μm of preswelling height (volume). Figure 2A illustrates the RVD process from the time-point where the cells achieve their MV to the end of hypotonic exposure. Cells concomitantly treated with MeHg (10 μM) fail to volume regulate and remain swollen throughout the experimental period. However, when Na^+ in the hypotonic buffer is replaced by N-methyl-D-glucamine (NMDG; 22 mM), volume regulation in the presence of MeHg occurs at near-normal rates (Fig. 2B), and is indistinguishable from controls (i.e., exposure to hypotonic buffer alone). In additional experiments, we have also measured ion (^{86}Rb, a marker for K^+), and amino acid (^{3}H-taurine, ^{3}H-aspartate) release on hypotonic induced swelling in the absence and presence of MeHg.

By combining volume measurements with intracellular ion measurements, one could determine not only the role of ions, but also how interference with crossmembrane ion movements impacts on volume regulation. We have calculated *(52)* that the uptake of $^{22}Na^+$ during the first 15 min of hypotonicity in the presence of MeHg approximates 537.2 ± 26.8 nmol/mg protein. Intracellular K^+ concentrations in primary astrocyte cultures are approx 130 mM. By assuming an average volume of 4 μL/mg protein, we obtain a K^+ content of 520 nmol K^+/mg protein. Our data show that in the presence of a hypotonic buffer and MeHg, 20% of the loaded ^{86}Rb is released from the cell during the 15-min exposure. Since ^{86}Rb release traces K^+, we can use the ^{86}Rb efflux to estimate K^+ and calculate an efflux of 104 nmol K^+/mg protein. In hypotonic buffer alone, 10% (52 nmol K^+/mg protein) of the preloaded ^{86}Rb is released. The increased uptake of Na^+ is more than sufficient to offset the increased K^+ (as ^{86}Rb) rate of efflux. The increased $^{22}Na^+$ influx seems to take place exclusively through activation of an amiloride sensitive Na^+/H^+ antiporter. The Na^+/H^+ transport system is known to be amiloride-sensitive and has been found in astrocytes. It is also interesting to note that influx of $^{22}Na^+$ is inhibited by amiloride, suggesting a specific site of action of MeHg. Preliminary data from our laboratory (Aschner et al., unpublished data) also suggest that the addition of

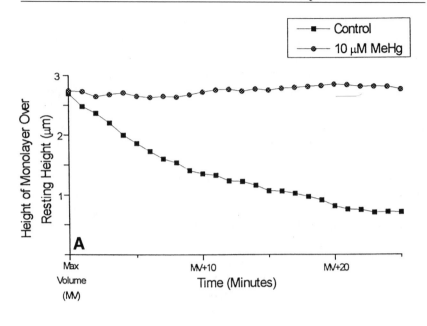

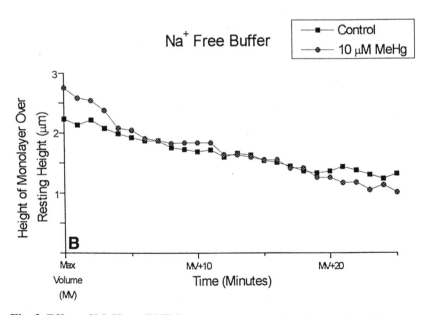

Fig. 2. Effect of MeHg on RVD in astrocytes exposed to hypotonic buffer. Rat primary astrocyte cultures were exposed to isotonic buffer for 15 min in the chamber, followed by hypotonic buffer ± 10 μ*M* MeHg for an additional 30 min.

amiloride to the hypotonic buffer completely reverses the MeHg-induced inhibition of RVD.

In summary, MeHg has been shown to cause astrocytic swelling in vitro and release of the preloaded [^{3}H] radiolabeled amino acids L-glutamate and D-aspartate *(48)*. This release is caused possibly by a swelling-induced mechanism, since it was inhibited by anion transport inhibitors in the same rank order (L-644,711 > SITS > furosemide) in which they inhibit hypotonic-induced swelling release of [^{3}H]-L-glutamate *(23)*. We also found that MeHg at 10 μ*M* totally inhibits uptake of these amino acids. Both these effects, namely increased release and decreased uptake, will serve to increase extracellular levels of these neurotoxic amino acids *(5)*, potentially leading to activation and overstimulation of neuronal *N*-methyl-D-aspartate (NMDA) receptors.

SUMMARY

In this chapter, astrocytic swelling, its mechanisms, and consequences have been briefly reviewed. It has been shown that astrocytic swelling is a frequent response to toxins *(2)*; it is associated with compromised energy metabolism, either owing to a direct effect of the toxins, or secondary to a failure of the supply of oxygen and substrates, such as in ischemia. As described in this chapter, astrocytic swelling leads to release of EAAs, and important homeostatic astrocytic functions are compromised, thus being likely to exacerbate the initial effects of the neurotoxins.

The electrical resistance technique offers an elegant means to study cellular mechanisms of swelling and RVD. When combined with the continuous perfusion method, it offers the added feature of release measurements of preloaded radiolabeled ions and amino acids. This is a promising assay system with great potential as an in vitro tool for the study of cytotoxicity. A modification of the existing chamber with suitable optics through the cell channel could also allow the simultaneous measurement of changes in intracellular ion concentrations using fluorescent probes. Thus, by combining volume measurements with intracellular ion measurements, one could not only determine the role of

---

MV occurred 3–5 min following exposure to hypotonic buffer. The figure represents RVD following MV (T = 18–20 min) after exposure to hypotonic buffer. **(A)** Cells exposed to hypotonic buffer swelled and then volume regulated to near-normal volume. Addition of 10 μ*M* MeHg completely inhibited RVD. **(B)** In the presence of Na$^+$-free buffer (replaced with NMDG), MeHg did not inhibit RVD. (Reprinted from ref. *52*, with kind permission from Elsevier Science-NL, Sara Burgerhartstraat 25, 1055 KV Amsterdam, The Netherlands.)

ions, such as Ca^{2+} or K^+, in RVD, but also determine how interference with such processes can impact on volume regulation and the release of endogenous substances.

In the experiments described herein, we examined swelling of confluent astrocytic monolayers on exposure to hypotonic solutions in the presence and absence of MeHg. This methodology is applicable to studying volume regulation not only in astrocytes, but any substratum-attached cell types, since most mammalian cell types, when exposed to hypotonic media, will swell and subsequently return to their normal volume. Furthermore, the technique can be utilized to screen chemicals that induce cell swelling and for the release of endogenous substances. With this method, it is not necessary to have a single confluent mono-layer of cells to study swelling and release, since both multilayers of cells or less than confluent cell cultures can be studied, although the system's sensitivity would change. Finally, from the economic point of view, the system is inexpensive compared to other cytotoxic screening methods. A lock-in amplifier can be purchased for approx $3000. The method is extremely reproducible and allows for many experiments to be run in a single day. Unlike many other methods, which offer a "snap-shot" in time, the electrical resistance technique combined with efflux measurements allows for continuous correlation of relative changes in cell volume and release of endogenous markers, allowing for sensitive measurements of cytotoxicity.

ACKNOWLEDGMENT

Support from NIH grants NIEHS 07331 and USEPA R-824087 to M. A. is gratefully acknowledged.

REFERENCES

1. Klatzo, I. Presidential address: neuropathological aspects of brain edema. J Neuro-pathol Exp Neurol 1967;26:1–13.
2. Kimelberg HK, Vitarella D, Aschner M. Effects of toxins on glia in relation to vasogenic and cytotoxic edema. In: Aschner M, Kimelberg HK, eds. The Role of Glia in Neurotoxicity. CRC, Boca Raton, FL, 1996, pp. 311–334.
3. Abbott NJ, ed. Glial–Neuronal Interactions. Ann NY Acad Sci 633. New York, 1991.
4. Kimelberg HK, Norenberg MD. Astrocytes. Sci Am 1989;260:66–76.
5. LoPachin R, Aschner M. Glial-neuronal interactions: the relevance to neurotoxic mechanisms. Toxicol Appl Pharmacol 1993;118:141–158.
6. Murphy S, ed. Astrocytes: Pharmacology and Function. Academic, New York, 1993.
7. Kimelberg HK, Aschner M. Astrocytes and their functions, past and present. In: Alcohol and Glial Cells. National Institute on Alcohol Abuse and Alcoholism Research Monograph, NIH Publication No. 94-3742, Bethesda, MD, Monograph 27, 1994, 1–40.

8. Kettenman H, Ransom B, eds. Astrocytes, 1996.
9. Aschner M, Kimelberg HK, eds. The Role of Glia in Neurotoxicity. CRC, Boca Raton, FL, 1996.
10. Jenkins LW, Povlishock JT, Becker DP, Miller JD, Sullivan HG. Complete cerebral ischemia: an ultrastructural study. Acta Neuropathol (Berlin) 1979;48:113–125.
11. Garcia JH. Experimental ischemic stroke: a review. Stroke 1984;15:5–14.
12. Bourke RS, Kimelberg HK, Daze M, Church G. Swelling and ion uptake in cat cerebrocortical slices: control by neurotransmitters and ion transport mechanisms. Neurochem Res 1983;8:5–24.
13. Kempski O, Staub F, Rosen FV, Zimmer M, Neu A, Baethmann A. Molecular mechanisms of glial swelling in vitro. Neurochem Pathol 1988;9:109–125.
14. Van Harreveld A, Fifkova E. Light and electron-microscopic changes in central nervous tissue after electrophoretic injection of glutamate. Exp Mol Pathol 1971;15:61–81.
15. Szatkowski M, Barbour B, Attwell D. Potassium-dependence of excitatory amino acid transport: resolution of a paradox. Brain Res 1991;555:343–345.
16. Walz W. Mechanism of rapid K^+-induced swelling of mouse astrocytes. Neurosci Lett 1992;135:243–246.
17. Barres BA, Chun LLY, Corey DP. Ion channels in vertebrate glia. Ann Rev Neurosci 1990;13:441–474.
18. Jalonen T. Single-channel characteristics of the large-conductance anion channel in rat cortical astrocytes in primary culture. Glia 1993;9:227–237.
19. Oliver CN, Stake-Reed PE, Stadtman ER, Liu GJ, Carney JM, Floyd RA. Oxidative damage to brain proteins, loss of glutamine synthetase activity and production of free radicals during ischemia/reperfusion-induced injury to gerbil brain. Proc Natl Acad Sci USA 1990;87:5144–5147.
20. Hall ED, Andrus PK, Yonkers PA. Brain hydroxyl radical generation in acute experimental head injury. J Neurochem 1993;60:588–594.
21. Hall ED, Braughler JM, McCall JM. Antioxidant effects in brain and spinal cord injury. J Neurotrauma 1992;9:S165–S172.
22. Choi DW, Rothman SM. The role of glutamate neurotoxicity in hypoxic-ischemic neuronal death. Annu Rev Neurosci 1990;13:171–182.
23. Kimelberg HK, Goderie SK, Higman S, Pang S, Waniewski RA. Swelling-induced release of glutamate, aspartate, and taurine from astrocyte cultures. J Neurosci 1990;10:1583–1591.
24. O'Connor ER, Kimelberg HK. Role of calcium in astrocyte volume regulation, ion and amino acid release. J Neurosci 1993;13:2638–2650.
25. Martin DL, Madelian V, Seligmann B, Shain W. The role of osmotic pressure and membrane potential in $K^{(+)}$-stimulated taurine release from cultured astrocytes and LRM55 cells. J Neurosci 1990;10:571–577.
26. Kimelberg HK, Frangakis MV. Furosemide- and bumetanide-sensitive ion transport and volume control in primary astrocyte cultures from rat brain. Brain Res 1985;361:125–134.
27. Olson JE, Sankar R, Holtzman D, James A, Fleischhacker D. Energy-dependent volume regulation in primary cultured cerebral astrocytes. J Cell Physiol 1986;128:209–215.
28. Pasantes-Morales H, Schousboe A. Volume regulation in astrocytes: a role for taurine as an osmoeffector. J Neurosci Res 1988;20:505–509.
29. Strange K, Emma F, Jackson P. Cellular and molecular physiology of volume-sensitive anion channels. Am J Physiol 1996;270:C711–C730.

30. Vitarella D, Kinelberg HK, Aschner M. Regulatory volume decrease in primary astrocyte cultures: relevance to methylmercury neurotoxicity. NeuroToxicology. 1996;17:117–123.

31. Vitarella D, DiRisio D, Kimelberg HK, Aschner M. Potassium and taurine release are highly correlated with regulatory volume decrease in neonatal primary rat astrocyte cultures. J Neurochem 1994;63:1143–1149.

32. Mountian I, Declercq PE, van Driessche W. Volume regulation in rat brain glial cells: Lack of substantial contribution of free amino acids. Am J Physiol 1996; 270:C1319–C1325.

33. Grinstein S, Dupre A, Rothstein A. Volume regulation by human lymphocytes—role of calcium. J Gen Physiol 1982;79:849–868.

34. Pierce SK, Politis AD. Ca^{2+}-activated cell volume recovery mechanisms. Ann Rev Physiol 1990;52:27–42.

35. Hoffmann EK, Kolb HA. Mechanisms of activation of regulatory volume responses after cell swelling. In: Gilles R, Hoffmann EK, Bolis L, eds. Comparative and Environmental Physiology, vol. 9. Springer-Verlag, New York, 1991, pp. 140–185.

36. Bender AS, Neary JT, Blicharska J, Norenberg L-OB, Norenberg MD. Role of calmodulin and protein kinase C in astrocytic cell volume regulation. J Neurochem 1992;58:1874–1882.

37. Gullans SR, Verbalis JG. Control of brain volume during hyperosmolar and hypoosmolar conditions. Ann Rev Med 1993;44:289–301.

38. Strange K, Morrison R. Volume regulation during recovery from chronic hypertonicity in brain glial cells. Am J Physiol 1992;263:C412–C419.

39. Cragoe EJ, Jr, Woltersdorf OW, Jr, Gould NP, Pietruszkiewicz AM, Ziegler C, Sakurai Y, et al. Agents for the treatment of brain edema. II. ((2,3,9,9a-tetrahydro-3-oxo-9a-substituted-1H-fluoren-7-yl)oxy) alkanoic acids and some of their analogues. J Med Chem 1986;29:825–841.

40. O'Connor ER, Kinelberg HK, Keese CR, Giaever I. Electrical impedance method for measuring volume changes in astrocytes. Am J Physiol 1993;264:C471–478.

41. Kimelberg HK, O'Connor ER, Sankar P, Keese C. Methods for determination of cell volume in tissue culture. Can J Physiol Pharmacol Suppl 1992;70:S323–S333.

42. Takeuchi T. Biological reactions and pathological changes in human beings and animals caused by organic mercury contamination. In: Hartung P, Dinman BD, eds. Environmental Mercury Contamination. Ann Arbor Science, Ann Arbor, MI, 1972, pp. 247–289.

43. Bakir F, Damluji SF, Amin-Zaki L, Murthada M, Khalidi A, Al-Rawi NY, et al. Methylmercury poisoning in Iraq. Science 1973;181:230–242.

44. Oyake Y, Tanaka M, Kubo H, Cichibu H. Neuropathological studies on organic mercury poisoning with special reference to the staining and distribution of mercury granules. Adv Neurol Sci 1966;10:744–750.

45. Garman RH, Weiss B, Evans HL. Alkylmercurial encephalopathy in the monkey; a histopathologic and autoradiographic study. Acta Neuropathol (Berlin) 1975; 32:61–74.

46. Charleston JS, Bolender RP, Mottet NK, Body RL, Vahter ME, Burbacher TM. Increases in the number of reactive glia in the visual cortex of *Macaca fascicularis* following subclinical long-term methyl mercury exposure. Toxicol Appl Pharmacol 1994;129:196–206.

47. Aschner M, Eberle N, Miller K, Kimelberg HK. Interaction of methylmercury with rat primary astrocyte cultures: effects on rubidium uptake and efflux and induction of swelling. Brain Res 1990;530:245–250.

48. Aschner M, Du Y-L, Gannon M, Kimelberg HK. Methylmercury-induced alterations in excitatory amino acid efflux from rat primary astrocyte cultures. Brain Res 1993;602:181–186.

49. Brookes N, Kristt DA. Inhibition of amino acid transport and protein synthesis by $HgCl_2$ and methylmercury in astrocytes: Selectivity and reversibility. J Neurochem 1989;53:1228–1237.

50. Dave V, Mullaney KJ, Goderie S, Kimelberg HK, Aschner M. Astrocytes as mediators of methylmercury (MeHg) neurotoxicity: Effects on D-aspartate and serotonin uptake. Dev Neurosci 1994;16:222–231.

51. Brookes N. *In vitro* evidence for the role of glutamate in the CNS toxicity of mercury. Toxicology 1992;76:245–256.

52. Vitarella D, Kimelberg HK, Aschner M. Inhibition of regulatory volume decrease (RVD) in swollen rat primary astrocyte cultures by methylmercury is due to increased amiloride-sensitive Na^+ uptake. Brain Res 1996;732:169–178.

4 Cytotoxicity Profiles for a Series of Investigational Compounds Using Liver Slice Technology and Human-Derived Cell Cultures

Sanjeev Thohan, PhD and Ho Chung, PhD

CONTENTS

INTRODUCTION
METHODS
RESULTS
DISCUSSION
ACKNOWLEDGMENT
REFERENCES

BACKGROUND

The use of in vitro screening in the development of new compounds has provided for the testing of compounds that cannot be safely studied in vivo in humans. Previous paradigms have employed test animal-based enzyme preparations or preneoplastic/neoplastic cell populations for evaluating candidate compounds *(1,2)*. Genetic alterations that result in neoplastic transformation can greatly alter the cellular responses. That is not to say that these cells do not have a utility, but that the altered sensitivity to chemical compounds may mask or enhance cytotoxicity end points, thus resulting in erroneous conclusions.

Normal human cells maintained in cell-culture conditions provide a testing paradigm that may be more appropriate for the assessment of cytotoxicity in vitro. Previous research efforts have employed end-point assays involving either dye activation or uptake, energy-dependent

From: *Toxicity Assessment Alternatives: Methods, Issues, Opportunities*
Edited by: H. Salem and S. A. Katz © Humana Press Inc., Totowa, NJ

substrate conversion, or radiolabeled precursor uptake *(3–5)*. These have provided great insight into cellular toxicity; however, the assays are technically delicate and not readily applicable to small numbers of cells. The Alamar blue cytotoxicity assay system provides an indicator that is a soluble nontoxic product, highly sensitive, stable in the culture medium, and suitable for normal cultured mammalian cells.

Since these isolated cell populations do not posses the complexity of a tissue, it was necessary to utilize an in vitro tissue preparation. Liver slice technology (LST) provides a paradigm that maintains the functional architecture of the tissue and provides metabolism profiles similar to those observed in vivo. It has been well established that cytotoxicity/target organ toxicity may arise from normal metabolic processes within the cell/tissue *(6,7)*. Drug metabolism-mediated toxicity may be envisioned as a balance of the mixed-function oxidase system and conjugation reactions. Reactive species may be products of phase I or phase II biotransformation. Alterations to the system may also result in net bioprotection or bioactivation by enhancement of inhibition of specific enzymes. The integrated use of in vitro systems to survey the target organ response has greatly increased the mechanistic understanding of drug metabolism and bioactivation. Cytotoxicity using cellular targets and the tissue slice system provide a versatile tool with which to probe the involvement of both the parent compound and metabolite(s) in the toxicity process.

Improvements in methodology of tissue slice generation and incubation have resulted in an increased use of tissue slices in the arenas of drug development and safety evaluation at the in vitro level *(8–11)*. From the area of liver slice investigations, experimental needs and final objectives have resulted in a wide variety of incubation techniques with relation to buffers, incubation conditions, and amounts of tissue to be used *(12)*. Using LST, the authors plan to probe and evaluate the utility of this technique in the assessment of investigational compound toxicity with the liver as a target organ. A series of model compounds and experimental candidates will be used for surveying the applicability of this type of in vitro toxicity screening as a simpler alternative to some of the conventionally used in vitro techniques. LST, by functional design, is readily applicable to a wide variety of species and may be adapted to other target tissues of interest *(13–15)*.

Based on the demonstrated metabolic capacity of LST, a system for the assessment of toxicity of known model compounds was initiated *(16)*. The research question to be examined was whether the liver slice system in tandem with cellular cytotoxicity using Alamar blue can provide a rapid in vitro assessment of toxicity. This necessitates the establishment of effect and no effect levels for rank ordering of toxicants. Initial parameters for the assessment of toxic insult were lactate dehydrogenase (cytosolic) and sorbitol dehydrogenase (mitochondrial) enzymes from liver slices. The release of these enzymes from the liver slice was used to generate an index of toxic insult as a result of exposure to a series of model toxicants. Growth index alteration was used to measure toxicity in the cell cultures. Model compounds having both in vitro and in vivo information concerning dose–toxicity relationships were used.

METHODS

Animals

Male Sprague Dawley Rats (180–220 g, Harlan Sprague Dawley, Indianapolis, IN) were utilized in this study. Phenobarbital was administered for three consecutive days via ip injection at 80 mg/kg. Saline was administered to the control groups. Rats were allowed food and water *ad libitum*. Animals were fasted overnight and prepared for terminal surgical anesthesia with pentobarbital (60 mg/kg). Livers were perfused with ice-cold 0.9% saline prior to excision.

Slice Preparation and Incubation

Livers were dissected into lobes and cores produced using a cylindrical stainless-steel corer (11.0-mm internal diameter) as outlined in Fig. 1. Cores of tissue were transferred to ice-cold 0.9% saline and slices generated immediately. A tissue core was loaded into the holder mechanism of the Krumdieck tissue slicer, and slices were generated by movement of the weighted tissue core over an oscillating razor blade. Tissue slices were swept away to a collection chamber by a stream of 0.9% saline (*see* Fig. 1). Using the tissue slicer in the above fashion, a slice was generated every 3–4 s. Slices were transferred to a shallow tray containing ice-cold 0.9% saline for selection and loading onto the incubation supports. Supports were then placed into 23-mL glass incubation vials containing 5 mL of Krebs-Henseleit buffer supplemented with 25 mM HEPES (pH 7.4) as demonstrated in Fig. 1.

Vials were then incubated horizontally in an enclosed Dynamic Organ Culture (DOC) incubator at 37 ± 0.5°C and rotated at 6 rpm (*see* Fig. 1). After the 1 h preincubation, vial inserts were transferred to vials containing fresh buffer medium and substrate. Lactate dehydrogenase (LDH; kit #228-50) and sorbitol dehydrogenase (SHD; kit #50-UV) were assayed using reagent kits from the Sigma Chemical Company (St. Louis, MO).

1. Core Preparation

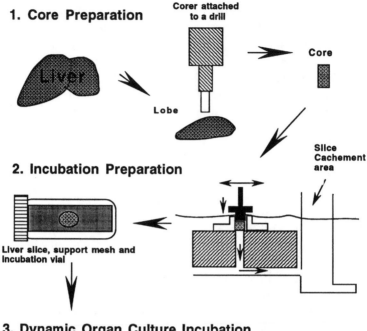

2. Incubation Preparation

3. Dynamic Organ Culture Incubation

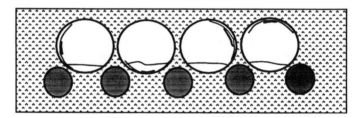

Fig. 1. Summary of the slice preparation and incubation procedure.

Microsomal Characterization

Tissue remnants from the core preparation will be used for the generation of subcellular fractions. Homogenates will be generated at 20% w/v by three bursts (5–10 s) of a polytron homogenizer (Brinkmann Instruments, Westbury, NY). Buffers and subsequent subcellular fractions were generated and stored according to the methods of Van der Hoeven and Coon *(17)* and Halpert et al. *(18)*, respectively. NADPH Cytochrome P450 reductase was quantified according to the method of Phillips and Langdon *(19)*. Cytochromes b5 and P450 were quantified according to Omura and Sato *(20,21)*. Microsomal UDP glucuronosyl transferase (UDPGT) was quantified according to Bock and White *(22)*.

Alkoxycoumarin Assay

The presence of free 7-hydroxycoumarin (7-HC; umbelliferone), i.e., unconjugated, was quantified using a Perkin Elmer LS5 Spectrofluorimeter (Norwalk, CT) at an excitation wavelength of 370 nm and emission wavelength of 450 nm as suggested by Greenlee and Poland *(23)*. Conjugates of the phase I metabolite, 7-HC, were determined by using specific hydrolytic enzymes. 7-Ethoxycoumain (7-EC) and 7-HC were obtained from the Sigma Chemical Company. Microsomal activities were assayed according to Matsubara et al. *(24)*. 7-Methoxycoumarin (7-MC) was obtained from the Aldrich Chemical Company (Milwaukee, WI). All other chemicals used were of the highest purity commercially available.

Cell Culture

Human aortic endothelial cells (HAEC), renal proximal tubule epithelial cells (RPTEC), and respective growth medium were obtained from the Clonetics Corporation (San Diego, CA). Cells from frozen stock were grown to confluence and working stock cultures generated. Growth characteristics were quantified using the Alamar blue reagent (Alamar Biosciences, Inc. Sacramento, CA). Alamar reagent was added aseptically at 10% volume of cells. The plates were then incubated at 37°C (5% CO_2) for designated time periods. The fluorescence of the Alamar dye was determined at an excitation wavelength of 485 nm and emission wavelength of 590 nm using a Microplate Fluorometer (Cambridge Technology, Inc., Watertown, MA). Results are expressed as either fluorescence units or fluorescence units normalized to respective control incubations (quadruplicate determinations). Investigational compounds were obtained from Sigma or from the Walter Reed Army Institute of Research (WRAIR, Washington, DC), and solubilized in dimethyl sulfoxide (DMSO). Investigational compounds were added to cell cultures such that the final concentration of DMSO in the incubation was <1%.

Statistics

Statistical evaluations were carried out using the Student's t test; $p < 0.10$ was considered to be significant.

RESULTS

Studies were initiated to compare effects of phenobarbital induction on the bioactivation profiles of a series of model and investigational compounds. In order to verify induction, subcellular fractions were generated from control and phenobarbital-pretreated rat livers. Tables 1 and 2

Table 1
Effects of Phenobarbital on Drug Metabolism Parameters
in Microsomal Fractions[a]

	Substrate, μM	Control	Phenobarbital
CYP450 reductase		80.8 ± 13.4	133.0 ± 36.9^{b}
(nmol/min/mg protein)			
Cyt b_5		0.49 ± 0.14	0.69 ± 0.14
(nmol/mg protein)			
CYP 450 content		0.71 ± 0.13	1.30 ± 0.24^{b}
(nmol/mg protein)			
7-MC	100	246 ± 80	763 ± 41^{b}
(pmol/min/mg protein)			
7-EC	100	268 ± 50	1114 ± 266^{b}
(pmol/min/mg protein)			
UDPGT activity	100	5.22 ± 0.67	7.63 ± 0.58^{b}
(nmol/min/mg protein)			

[a]$n = 6$ rats/treatment.
[b]Denotes significantly different from controls ($p < 0.10$).

Table 2
Comparison of Microsomal and Liver Slice Metabolism
Parameters in Response to Phenobarbital Pretreatment In Vivo[a]

	Control	Phenobarbital
CYP450 reductase	1.6	
Cyt b_5	1.4	
CYP 450 content	1.8	
7-MC activity	3.1	3.3
7-EC activity	4.1	5.3
UDPGT activity	1.5	1.2

[a]All values are fold increase over control (PB/con). Microsomal
preparations from the same tissue as the liver slices. UDPGT assay in
microsomes used 4-MU (4-Methylumbelliferone) and LST 7-HC
(Umbelliferone).

provide a summary of the findings with phenobarbital pretreatment.
Microsomal metabolism was quantified using alkoxycoumarin derivatives. Both the slice and microsomal substrate concentrations were at
100 μM. The subcellular fractions were generated from the remnant
tissues from liver slice preparation. Increases effected by phenobarbital
pretreatment were found to be consistent with previously reported values. Table 2 presents a summary of the induction profiles. Similar quali-

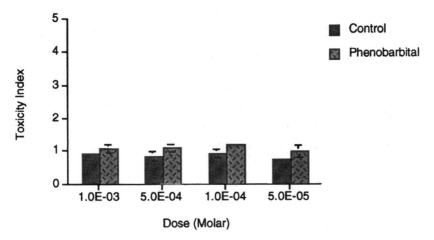

Fig. 2. Toxicity assessment of acetaminophen using LDH release from rat liver slices. Toxicity index used in this presentation is a factor generated from the percent of enzyme released in treatment groups normalized to vehicle controls in LST. ($n = 3$; each study using pooled slices from 3 rats; mean ± SEM.)

tative effects were seen in both the slice and microsomal investigations. This correlation showed that the slice system responds in a manner similar to that in alternative in vitro techniques. In fact, the greater fold-induction seen with 7-EC metabolism may be owing to the physiological barriers posed by the architecture of the liver slice system vs the nonrestricted enzyme access offered in the microsomal incubation. It was not technically possible to determine the specific content of the slice CYP 450 and reductase. However, it is possible to calculate these contents in slices based on slice protein and microsomal recoveries from subcellular fractionation.

The toxicity profiles from the various compounds tested may be found in Figs. 2–12. The toxicity index used in this presentation is a factor generated from the percent of enzyme released in treatment groups normalized to vehicle controls in LST. Consequently, values that are in the vicinity of 1 (one) on the toxicity index are indicative of little or no toxicity. These studies provide a framework within which to create a database of information, such that compounds may be ranked with regard to toxicity potential via bioactivation. No overt toxicity was noted by the release of LDH from the liver slices in both the control and phenobarbital-pretreated rat liver slices when exposed to varying concentrations of acetaminophen or paraquat (*see* Figs. 2 and 4, respectively). However there was a significant dose-dependent increase in the toxicity to the mitochondria, as measured by increased release of SDH from the liver

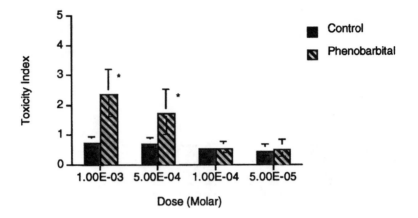

Fig. 3. Toxicity assessment of acetaminophen using SDH release from rat liver slices. Toxicity index used in this presentation is a factor generated from the percent of enzyme released in treatment groups normalized to vehicle controls in LST. ($n = 2$; each study using slices from 3 rats; mean ± SEM. *Denotes significantly different from control value at $p < 0.10$.)

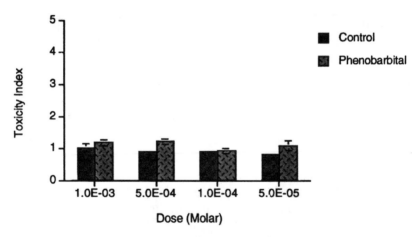

Fig. 4. Toxicity assessment of paraquat using LDH release from rat liver slices. Toxicity Index used in this presentation is a factor generated from the percent of enzyme released in treatment groups normalized to vehicle controls in LST. ($n = 3$; each study using pooled slices from 3 rats; mean ± SEM.)

slices form phenobarbital-pretreated rats using both acetaminophen and paraquat (*see* Figs. 3 and 5, respectively). Acetaminophen toxicity was noted only at concentrations >0.5 mM. All concentrations (from 50 μM to 1 mM) of the paraquat-exposed liver slices from phenobarbital-pretreated rats demonstrated a significant release of SDH. In fact, there was

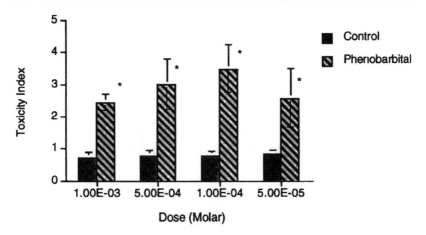

Fig. 5. Toxicity assessment of paraquat using SDH release from rat liver slices. Toxicity index used in this presentation is a factor generated from the percent of enzyme released in treatment groups normalized to vehicle controls in LST. ($n = 2$; each study using slices from 3 rats; mean ± SEM. *Denotes significantly different from control value at $p < 0.10$.)

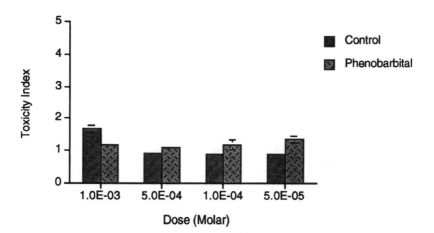

Fig. 6. Toxicity assessment of primaquine using LDH release from rat liver slices. Toxicity Index used in this presentation is a factor generated from the percent of enzyme released in treatment groups normalized to vehicle controls in LST. ($n = 3$; each study using pooled slices from 3 rats; mean ± SEM.)

no noted difference in the amount of SDH released at any of the concentrations investigated for paraquat. It seemed as though there was a quantal response to the release of SDH from the phenobarbital-pretreated liver slice. Primaquine-associated toxicity was primarily of mitochon-

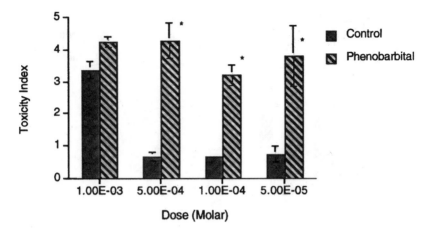

Fig. 7. Toxicity assessment of primaquine using SDH release from rat liver slices. Toxicity Index used in this presentation is a factor generated from the percent of enzyme released in treatment groups normalized to vehicle controls in LST. ($n = 2$; each study using slices from 3 rats; mean ± SEM. *Denotes significantly different from control value at $p < 0.10$.)

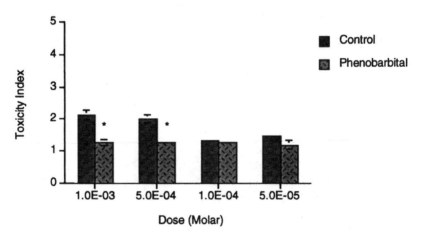

Fig. 8. Toxicity assessment of WR238605AC using LDH release from rat liver slices. Toxicity index used in this presentation is a factor generated from the percent of enzyme released in treatment groups normalized to vehicle controls in LST. ($n = 3$; each study using pooled slices from 3 rats; mean ± SEM. *Denotes significantly different from control value at $p < 0.10$.)

drial origin. At the millimolar concentration, there was a significant amount of toxicity as indicated by LDH and SDH release (*see* Figs. 6 and 7). However, this toxicity was found to be dose-dependent in the

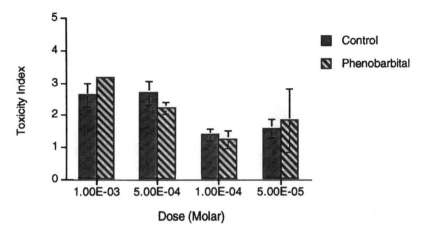

Fig. 9. Toxicity assessment of WR238605AC using SDH release from rat liver slices. Toxicity index used in this presentation is a factor generated from the percent of enzyme released in treatment groups normalized to vehicle controls in LST. ($n = 2$; each study using slices from 3 rats; mean $\pm$ SEM.)

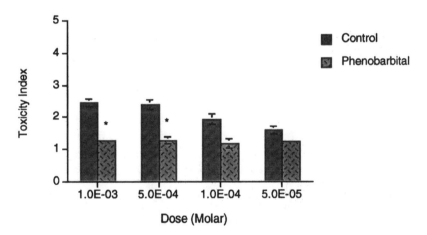

Fig. 10. Toxicity assessment of WR242511AE using LDH release from rat liver slices. Toxicity Index used in this presentation is a factor generated from the percent of enzyme released in treatment groups normalized to vehicle controls in LST. ($n = 3$; each study using pooled slices from 3 rats; mean $\pm$ SEM. *Denotes significantly different from control value at $p < 0.10$.)

control rat liver slice incubations. Rat liver slices from phenobarbital-pretreated rats provided a more interesting profile for primaquine exposure. There was a shift in the site of toxic insult from the parenchymal membrane to the mitochondrial membrane as indicated by the different

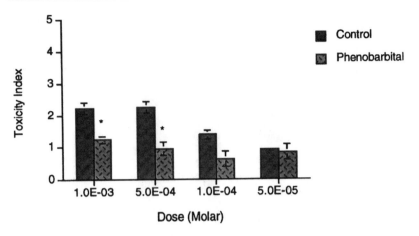

Fig. 11. Toxicity assessment of WR006026AF using LDH release from rat liver slices. Toxicity index used in this presentation is a factor generated from the percent of enzyme released in treatment groups normalized to vehicle controls in LST. ($n = 3$; each study using pooled slices from 3 rats; mean± SEM. *Denotes significantly different from control value at $p < 0.10$.)

patterns of enzyme release. In the 1.0-mM incubations, there was a 25% decrease in LDH release from the in the phenobarbital-pretreated liver slices as compared with control liver slices. Alternatively, primaquine was determined to be highly toxic to the mitochondria at all concentrations tested in phenobarbital-pretreated liver slices. A quantal release of SDH was observed using phenobarbital-pretreated liver slices exposed to primaquine. This was similar to the observation with the use of paraquat as a test article for toxicity assessment. Significant differences were noted between control and phenobarbital-pretreated slices at concentrations below 1.0 mM.

Using the investigational compound WR238605AC, LDH release was found to follow a shallow dose-dependent increase in toxicity (*see* Fig. 8). Significant differences were found at the 0.5- and 1.0-mM concentrations between control incubations. There was a 35–40% decrease in LDH release from the phenobarbital-pretreated slices on comparison to controls. These significant differences were noted at the 0.5- and 1.0-mM doses. WR238605AC was found to be equi-toxic at all concentrations tested in either treatment group, as measured by SDH release (*see* Fig. 9).

Figures 10 and 11 are preliminary results that demonstrate similar trends in the dose-dependent release of LDH from control liver slices. WR006026AF showed significant differences between concentrations

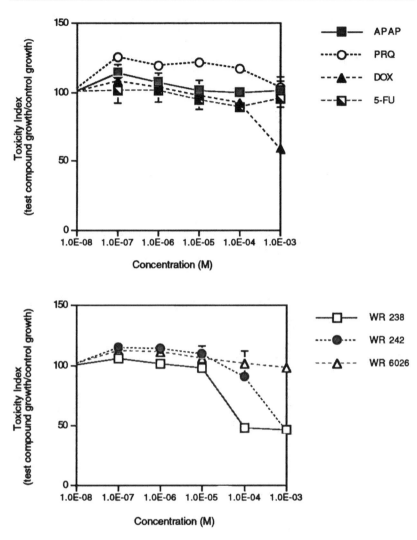

Fig. 12. Renal proximal tubule epithelial cellular toxicity assay. Data presented are typical results presented as mean ± SD from quadruplicate incubations.

below 100 µ*M* and concentrations of 0.5 and 1.0 m*M* (*see* Fig. 11). There was a trend toward increasing release of LDH as may be readily seen from control liver slices; however, there was no significant difference found between concentrations for WR242511AE (Fig. 10). In both cases, there were significant differences between control and phenobarbital-pretreatment groups at the 0.5- and 1.0-m*M* concentrations. Phenobarbital pretreatment effected a 40–50% decrement in the release of

LDH. Using phenobarbital-pretreated liver slices, there was no difference in toxicity index noted between vehicle controls and the treatment at various concentrations. There was no statistical significance noted between concentration groups of the phenobarbital-pretreated rat liver slice incubations.

The results in Fig. 12 represent the mean and standard deviation from quadruplicate incubations of an initial seeding density of 2000 cells/mL. Acetaminophen (APAP), Primaquine (PRQ), and 5-Fluorouracil (5-FU) were determined to be nontoxic at doses from the μM to mM range. Dox was found to be mildly toxic above the 100-μM doses. These observations show that APAP does not have a parent compound-associated toxicity. The Walter Reed (WR) series of compounds produced a dose-dependent toxicity. The LD_{50} equivalent ranking was found to be separated by a 10-fold difference in toxic dose, i.e., 10 μM for WR238605AC and 100 μM for WR242511AE. WR006026AF did not produce an inhibition of growth in the RPTEC.

DISCUSSION

From our studies, characteristic induction of drug-metabolizing enzymes by phenobarbital was confirmed. An advantage of using LST to perform bioactivation studies is the ability to prepare subcellular fractions from the same tissue. This allows for the quantification of drug-metabolizing enzymes in the absence of an *in situ* methodology. This property of the system will allow for the determination of specific isoform involvement and, thus, increase the understanding of the mechanism behind the toxicity. Additionally, the use of specific metabolic enhancers or inhibitors in both LST and subcellular fractions could produce a profile that would shed light onto which isoforms are major contributors in the bioactivation of a candidate compound.

Increases in the hepatic *O*-demethylase, *O*-deethylase, and glucuronosyl transferase activities were found to correlate well between microsomes and liver slices, thus suggesting that the LST responds in a similar manner to the in vivo situation and that patterns of drug metabolism are consistent with established in vitro methods of study. There was, however, a greater induction observed using 7-EC as a substrate. This represents a paradigm shift from saturating conditions that are present in the microsomal metabolism incubation to one of physiological barriers. In the microsomal incubation, the conditions are maximized such that concentrations of cofactors and substrates are saturating. Microsomal incubation allows for measurement of maximal rates of metabolism. It was decided to use similar concentrations to facilitate metabolism profile/rate comparisons. In the liver slice incubation, there are physiological barriers that provide compartmental metabolism. The metabolism is dependent on the uptake of parent compound and release of the metabolite into the medium. Additionally, the cofactor supply for drug metabolism is wholly dependent on intermediary metabolism. This feature closely replicates the *in situ* situation on comparison to subcellular fractions and isolated cell populations.

Using the LST system, we established metabolism/toxicity profiles that were consistent with previous findings in other in vitro systems with respect to paraquat and acetaminophen using control rat liver slices. However, the toxicity to the mitochondrial membrane as indicated by the increase in release of SDH may represent a new finding. An alteration in the integration between phase I and phase II may be contributory to the toxicity observed. The utility of this system was demonstrated in an initial survey of the investigational WR series of compounds. These compounds demonstrated toxicity at millimolar concentrations using both LDH and SDH as indicators of toxic insult in control rat liver slices. There was a dose-dependent reduction in the release of enzymes from the liver slices. Osmotic and oncotic changes were not considered to be significant contributing factors to the enzyme release seen.

Phenobarbital pretreatment provided a shift in the site of toxic insult from the membrane to the mitochondria in acetaminophen, paraquat, and primaquine studies. These results suggest that the induction of drug metabolism may have produced an imbalance in metabolite homeostasis. From alkoxycoumarin studies done previously in this laboratory, it was found that phenobarbital induction produced a higher amount of unconjugated (free) 7-HC from 7-MC and 7-EC *(16)*. This was taken to show the lag of phase II behind phase I metabolism in integrated metabolism. As may be expected, if the toxic moiety is not conjugated, there may be an elaboration of toxicity. This underscores the need for marker substrate analyses to be performed in tandem with toxicity investigations. These marker substrates not only allow for the characterization of alterations to specific isoforms, but also provide an indication of the overall integration of drug metabolism. In the absence of specific metabolite information from the candidate compounds, the likely toxicant would be a result of phase I metabolism. It is well established that the toxicities of acetaminophen and paraquat arise from the formation of quinone-like compounds that undergo redox cycling. Phenobarbital is known to increase the capacity of phase II glucuronidation and glutathione transferases. However, as seen from the marker alkoxycoumarin data, there is a lag in the integration of metabolism in time and capacity. Furthermore, there was a greater induction of phase I metabolism over the phase II metabolism. Studies to examine alterations in glutathione conjugation in noninduced and induced rat liver slices are currently in progress.

Phenobarbital pretreatment showed a decrease in the level of toxic insult to parenchymal cell membranes by the WR series of compounds as indicated by a significant reduction in the release of LDH from the liver slices. Completion of the SDH release profile will provide additional information with which to create a ranking of toxicity. These observations from LDH and limited SDH release studies may be interpreted as a "bioprotection" by pretreatment with phenobarbital. The mechanism behind this may be examined by metabolite analysis from the slice incubate medium. The metabolite profile on comparison with untreated liver slice incubations will delineate whether there are alterations in the rate of metabolism of an alternative pathway that are responsible for the results seen. These observations emphasize the need to understand the balance between phase I and phase II metabolism.

These preliminary cell-culture studies provide a framework within which to conduct more in-depth studies. Renal endothelial cells were chosen as representative cells that are metabolically inert with respect to drug metabolism. This will allow for the detection of parent compound-based toxicity. These cell cultures are from a normal human origin and would therefore more closely represent the *in situ* situation for short-term assays. As mentioned earlier, it is possible to incorporate cells of a tumorigenic origin; however, genetic alterations in the tumorigenic process could introduce variables to skew the results.

RPTEC provided stable and reproducible growth patterns with good sensitivity. Initial plating densities of 250 cells/well could be distinguished from the background of the RPTEC cultures. A doubling time of approx 24 h was found to be in agreement with the manufacturer's claims. Control test compounds were chosen based on their reported toxicity in a variety of in vitro test systems. However, using the RPTEC, there was no significant toxic response observed. In some cases, there was the suggestion that the presence of the test compound was enhancing the cellular growth. In all cases, the fluorescent signal was corrected for vehicle background. Furthermore, a toxicity index was generated for each compound by normalizing to a control incubation. In some cases, there was a variability that produced a standard deviation larger than the symbol. These are preliminary studies, and consequently, some of these systematic errors will be eliminated in future studies.

As may be readily appreciated from the results, there is a need for further optimization with respect to cell density. The apparent leveling off of the dose–response curve at 50% inhibition for WR238605AC and

WR242511AE may be owing to compound solubility. These candidate compounds are highly hydrophobic and require solubilization in a DMSO carrier vehicle. Studies were conducted to determine the maximal content of DMSO in order to achieve higher test compound concentrations. DMSO content of >1% was found to inhibit cellular growth significantly. It may also be that the concentration per cell unit is not optimized for maximal inhibition. Studies are currently under way to investigate and optimize these variables. Future studies will involve the use of a battery of test compounds with a series of human cell cultures such that a rank ordering of toxic potential may be achieved.

It should not be taken that these assay systems will replace in vivo animal testing, but rather that they will supplement the research efforts for faster movement of candidate drugs for preclinical development. Surveying large numbers of compounds for toxicity prioritization would be more prudent in a cell-culture situation where the environment is clearly defined and less expensive. Furthermore, judicious use of the tissue slice system may result in the reduction of the number of test animals in the early stages of drug development. This in turn will provide significant savings in time, money, and hours of labor.

ACKNOWLEDGMENT

The authors would like to recognize the invaluable assistance of David Petullo in this research effort.

REFERENCES

1. Ames BN, Durston WE, Yamasaki E, Lee FD. Carcinogens are mutagens: A simple test system combining liver homogenates for activation and bacteria for detection. Proc Natl Acad Sci USA 1973;70:2281.
2. Grisham JW, Smith GJ. Predictive and mechanistic evaluation of toxic responses in mammalian cell culture systems. Pharmacol Rev 1984;36:151S.
3. Weisenthal LM, Marsden JA, Dill PL, Malcuso CK. A novel dye exclusion method for testing in vitro chemosensitivity of novel human tumors. Cancer Res 1983;43:749.
4. Page M, Bejaoui N, Cinq Mars B, Lemieux P. Optimization of the tetrazolium assay for the measurement of cell number and cytotoxicity. Int J Immunopharmacol 1988;10:785.
5. Wemme H, Pfeifer S, Heck R, Muller-Quernheim J. Measurement of lymphocyte proliferation: Critical analysis of radioactive and photometric methods. Immunobiology 1992;185:79.
6. Conney AH. Induction of microsomal P-450 enzymes: the first Bernard Brodie lecture at Pennsylvania State University. Life Sci 1986;39:2493.
7. Guengerich FP. Reactions and significance of cytochrome P-450 enzymes. J Biol Chem 1991;266:10,019.
8. Krumdieck CL, Dos Santos JE, Ho K. A new instrument for the rapid preparation of tissue slices. Anal Biochem 1983;104:118.

9. Smith PF, Gandolfi AJ, Krumdieck CL, Putnam CW, Zukoski CF, Davis WM, et al. Dynamic Organic Culture of precision cut liver slices for in vitro toxicology. Life Sci 1985;36:1367.

10. Sipes IG, Fisher RL, Smith PF, Stine ER, Gandolfi AJ, Brendel K. A dynamic liver culture system: A tool for studying chemical biotransformation and toxicity. Mech Models Toxicol 1987;11:20.

11. Azri S, Gandolfi AJ, Brendel K. Precision-cut liver slices: an in vitro system for profiling hepatotoxicants. In Vitro Toxicol 1990;3:309.

12. Fisher RL, Shaugnessy RP, Jenkins PM, Austin ML, Roth GL, Gandolfi AJ, Brendel K. Dynamic organ culture is superior to multiwell plate culture for maintaining precision-cut tissue slices. Optimization of tissue culture, part 1. Toxicol methods 1995;5:99–113.

13. Barr J, Weir AJ, Brendel K, Sipes IG. Liver slices in dynamic organ culture I: an alternative *in vitro* technique for the study of rat hepatic drug metabolism Xenobiotica 1990;21:331.

14. Barr J, Weir AJ, Brendel K, Sipes IG. Liver slices in dynamic organ culture II: an *in vitro* cellular technique for the study of integrated drug metabolism using human tissue. Xenobiotica 1990;21:341.

15. Kane AS, Thohan S. Dynamic culture of fish hepatic tissue slices to assess phase I and phase II biotransformation. Techniques in Aquatic Toxicology. CRC, Boca Raton, FL, 1996, pp. 37–39.

16. Thohan S, Chung H, Weiner M. Liver slices in dynamic organ culture (LSDOC) as a model system for integrated phase I–phase II drug metabolism. Toxicologist 1995;34:1524.

17. Van der Hoeven TA, Coon MJ. Preparation and properties of partially purified cytochrome P-450 and reduced NADPH P-450 reductase from rabbit liver microsomes. J Biol Chem 1974;249:6102.

18. Halpert J, Nausland B, Betman B. Suicide inactivation of rat liver cytochrome P-450 by chloramphenicol *in vivo* and *in vitro*. Mol Pharmacol 1983;21:445.

19. Phillips AH, Langdon RG. Hepatic triphosphopyridine nucleotide cytochrome c reductase: Isolation, characterization and kinetic studies. J Biol Chem 1962; 237:2652.

20. Omura T, Sato R. The carbon monoxide-binding pigment of liver microsomes. I. Evidence for its hemoprotein nature. J Biol Chem 1964;239:2370.

21. Omura T, Sato R. The carbon-monoxide binding pigment. II. solubilization, purification and properties. J Biol Chem 1964;239:2379.

22. Bock KW, White IAH. UDP-glucuronosyltransferase in perfused rat liver and in microsomes: influence of Phenobarbital and 3-methylcholanthrene. Eur J Biochem 1974;46:451.

23. Greenlee WF, Poland A. An improved assay of ethoxycoumarin O-deethylase activity. J Pharmacol Exp Ther 1977;205:596.

24. Matsubara T, Otsubo S, Yoshihara E, Touchi A. Biotransformation of coumarin derivatives (2) oxidative metabolism of 7-alkoxycoumarin by microsomal enzymes and a simple procedure for 7-alkoxycoumarin dealkylase. Jpn J Pharmacol 1982;33:41.

5 Antagonistic Interaction of Sodium Arsenite and Lead Sulfate with UV Light on Sister Chromatid Exchanges in Human Peripheral Lymphocytes

Spiros P. Katsifis, PhD
and Patrick L. Kinney, PhD

CONTENTS

INTRODUCTION
MATERIALS AND METHODS
RESULTS
DISCUSSION
REFERENCES

INTRODUCTION

Several metals have been found to be mutagenic and carcinogenic in humans and experimental animals *(1–3)*. Epidemiological studies have shown that nickel is carcinogenic in humans as well as in animals *(1,2)*. Human as well as animal carcinogenicity studies, chromosomal aberrations, and morphological transformation in Syrian hamster embryo cells (SHE) indicate that Pb(II) may be a weak carcinogen *(3–5)*. Epidemiological studies have shown that inorganic arsenic exposure can cause cancer of the skin and lung *(6)*. However, reliable indications from animal mutagenic or carcinogenic studies are lacking *(7)*.

Although able data indicate that several metals are carcinogenic, their modes of action and their molecular mechanisms have not been fully elucidated *(2,3)*. Several epidemiological studies utilize cytogenetic and molecular markers to identify exposure to carcinogenic agents

From: *Toxicity Assessment Alternatives: Methods, Issues, Opportunities*
Edited by: H. Salem and S. A. Katz © Humana Press Inc., Totowa, NJ

(8,9). Among the most widely used biomarkers to identify exposure to genotoxic agents is the induction of sister chromatid exchange (SCE) *(10–12)*.

Ni(II), As(III), Pb(II), and UV light are inducers of SCEs *(2,7,13–18)*. Sodium arsenite has been found to increase the SCE frequency in human lymphocytes and mammalian cells. An additive effect was observed with a combined treatment of low doses of UV light and sodium arsenite in CHO cells *(7)*, but this metal does not affect the yield of diepoxybutane- (DEB) induced SCEs in human lymphocytes *(19)*. Lead has been reported to induce SCE in human lymphocytes *(15,16)*, but in other mammalian cells, the increase in SCE frequency was not statistically significant *(5,20)*. Pb(II) in V79 cells enhances significantly the number of UV light-induced SCEs *(20)*.

The synergistic interaction of nickel with DNA-damaging agents, such as B(a)P, UV light, and X-rays, in SHE has also been reported *(21)*. The mutagenic activity of Cr(VI) has been found to be enhanced by Ni(II) in the Chinese hamster HGPRT assay *(22)*. Lead compounds have been reported to enhance viral transformation of SHE cells *(23)* and the number of tumors in animals induced by some organic compounds *(24)*. Environmental exposures to arsenicals have been correlated with an increased risk of skin cancer among human populations exposed to high levels of sunlight *(25)*. However, epidemiological studies in people exposed to the metal report no difference in the induction of SCEs or chromosomal aberrations (CAs) compared to the untreated controls *(26)*. UV light enhances mutagenesis and SCE induction by nickel *(22)*.

Recently we reported that the treatment of cultured human blood lymphocytes with relatively low doses of $NiSO_4$ produced a significant increase in the SCE frequencies over the control. Nevertheless, combined treatment of $NiSO_4$ and UV light, X-rays, or Cr(VI) produced an antagonistic effect *(17,27)*.

For the present studies, we selected three metals with the common feature of interference with normal DNA replication or repair processes and failure to produce significant levels of DNA damage *(1,2)*. Interference with normal DNA replication or with replication occurring during DNA repair may enhance the biological activity of other classes of carcinogens. Comutagenic and cocarcinogenic activity has been reported for all three metals *(2,7,20,25)*.

The purpose of this study was to investigate whether the selected metals [Pb(II), As(III)] are capable of inducing SCEs in human lymphocytes and to assess the interaction of these metals with UV-light for the formation of SCEs.

MATERIALS AND METHODS

Cell Culture and Treatment

Different concentrations of $NaAsO_2$ and $PbSO_4$ (Fisher Scientific, Pittsburgh, PA) were used alone or in combination with UV light (200 ergs/mm^2). Fresh solutions of each compound were prepared on the day of each experiment. Thirty milliliters of peripheral blood were obtained in heparinized vacutainers from normal, nonsmoking subjects between the ages of 25 and 40 who had no history of exposure to heavy metals or any other DNA-damaging agent. This was accomplished by questionnaires given to each donor (28). At least two human subjects were analyzed for each experiment. Zero point eight milliliters of blood (5.5 × 10^6 leukocytes) was added to RPMI-1640 media supplemented with 10% fetal bovine serum, 100 U/mL penicillin, and 100 µg/mL streptomycin. Twenty milligrams per milligram of phytohemagglutinin (PHA), different concentrations of the experimental metal, and 20 µg/mL bromodeoxyuridine (BrdU) were added just before incubation. The final volume was adjusted to 10 mL in each of the cultured flasks with medium. All reagents for the cell-culture medium, PHA, and BrdU were obtained from Sigma Chemical Company (St. Louis, MO). The flasks were protected from light to prevent photolysis of substituted DNA by BrdU and were incubated with tightened caps at 37°C for 68.5 h (12). At 66 h of incubation, 0.08 µg/mL of Colcemid (Gibco-BRL, Gaithersburg, MD) was added to each flask, and they were returned to the incubator for another 2.5 h (17).

After 68.5 h of incubation, the flasks were slightly shaken, the contents were centrifuged, and the supernatant was discarded. Then the cells were treated with a 75-mM KCl hypotonic solution and centrifuged. The supernatant was discarded, and the remaining cells were fixed, three times, with methanol:acetic acid (3:1, v/v). From a suspension of the fixed cells, slides were prepared and stained with Giemsa. The slides were coded and randomly scored by a team of two scorers. Twenty to 30 well-spread, second-division metaphases with distinct differential staining of SCEs were scored for each treatment with a maximum of 15 cells from any one slide.

UV Light Irradiation

Aliquots of 0.80 mL of whole human blood were transferred to 40-mm diameter Petri dishes, and irradiated (in open dishes) with UV light of short wavelength (~254 nm) using an incidence dose rate at the irradiated surface of 20 ergs/mm^2/s. The energy flux was measured with a short-wave meter (Model J-225, Ultra-Violet Products, San Gabriel, CA).

Statistical Methods

The statistical significance for SCE induced by the individual treatments of Ni(II), Pb(II), As(III), or UV light were determined by Dunnett's test. To evaluate the significance of the interaction factor (IF), a 95% confidence interval was calculated *(17)*.

To investigate the interaction between Ni(II), Pb(II), and As(III) with UV light, for the induction of SCEs, we used the following formula *(17)*.

$$IF = (GM - \text{Control}) - [(G - \text{Control}) + (M - \text{Control})]$$
$$= GM - G - M + \text{Cont}$$

where IF is the interaction factor; G the mean SCE response to genotoxic agent (UV light); M the mean SCE response to metal (Ni[II], Pb[II], As[III]); GM means the mean SCE response to combined treatment; and Control means the mean SCE response under control conditions. A positive IF denotes synergy, a negative IF denotes antagonism, and a zero IF denotes additivity *(17)*.

RESULTS

Peripheral human lymphocytes were treated with $NiSO_4$, $PbSO_4$, or $NaAsO_2$ and UV light, and the induction of SCE was determined with each metal alone and in combination with a UV light *(13,27)*. Ni(II) induced SCEs between 5 and 50 μM in a dose-dependent fashion with a decrease at 100 μM. $PbSO_4$ induced a low, but significant level of SCEs, with a plateau in the response above 1000 μM. Arsenite produced the greatest increase in SCE frequency with a range of 7.1–16.20 SCE/cell. Analysis of variance (ANOVA) and tests of significance (Dunnett's, 95% CI) were performed for all SCE values. All the tests for the treatments of metal salts, UV light, or the combined treatments of metal and UV light were found to be significant at the 0.05 level or greater compared to the untreated control. These results are in agreement with the findings of other workers for similar treatments of human lymphocytes with the same metal salts *(5,15,16,18,22)*.

The combined treatment of Ni(II) and UV light induced SCE frequencies ranging from 7.77 SCE/cell to 11.64 SCE/cell, and those induced by the Ni(II) treatment alone ranged from 7.80 SCE/cell to 11.00 SCE/cell *(13,27)*. The IF ranged from –0.80 to –3.02 (Table 1).

For the combined treatments of the three lowest concentrations of Pb(II) with UV light the SCE frequencies ranged from 9.15 to 10.58 SCE/cell *(13)*. At the highest Pb(II) treatment in combination with UV light, the frequency of SCEs was less (8.02 SCE/cell) compared to Pb(II) treatment alone (8.71 SCE/cell) with a negative IF (Table 2). The

Table 1
NiSO$_4$ + UV Light[a]

Treatment[b]	Metal, μM	IF ± SE$_{IF}$[c]	95% CI of IF
200 ergs/mm^2 + NiSO$_4$	05	−2.64 ± 0.97	−4.56, −0.72[d]
	10	−0.80 ± 1.04	−2.86, 1.26
	25	−3.02 ± 1.06	−5.12, −0.92[d]
	50	−1.97 ± 0.98	−3.91, −0.03[d]
	100	−2.40 ± 1.00	−4.38, −0.42[d]

[a]After ref. *(27)*.
[b]Whole-blood cultures were set from two human subjects for the metal combined with UV light treatment.
[c]Tests of significance were performed for the IF.
[d]IF significant at 95% CI. A positive IF denotes synergy, a negative IF denotes antagonism, and a zero IF denotes antagonism.

Table 2
PbSO$_4$ + UV Light

Treatment[a]	NiSO$_4$, μM	IF ± SE$_{IF}$[b]	95% CI of IF
200 ergs/mm^2 + PbSO$_4$	250	−0.44 ± 0.76	−1.94, 1.06
	500	−0.85 ± 0.73	−2.29, 0.59
	1000	−0.36 ± 0.86	−2.06, 1.34
	2000	−2.99 ± 0.81	−4.59, −1.39[c]

[a]Whole-blood cultures were set from two human subjects for the metal combined with UV light treatments.
[b]Tests of significance were performed for the IF.
[c]IF significant at 95% CI. A positive IF denotes synergy, a negative IF denotes antagonism, and a zero IF denotes additivity.

combined treatments of the three lowest concentrations of Pb(II) with UV light exerted no antagonistic effect ($p > 0.05$) (Table 2). However, at the highest concentration of Pb(II) combined with UV light, a significant antagonistic response was observed (Table 2). Furthermore, for most of the combined treatments, the frequency of SCE was approximately additive (Table 2).

For the combined treatments of the three lowest concentrations of As(III) with UV light, the SCE frequencies ranged from 8.76 to 11.91 SCE/cell, and for the As(III) treatment alone from 7.10 to 11.47 SCE/cell *(13)*. At the highest As(III) concentration tested, the frequency of SCE was higher (16.17 SCE/cell) compared to the combined treatments of the same metal concentration with UV light (10.94 SCE/cell). However, most of the combined treatments of As(III) with UV light produced a negative IF (Table 3).

Table 3
$NaAsO_2$ + UV Light

Treatment[a]	$NaAsO_2$, μM	$IF \pm SE_{IF}$[b]	95% CI of IF
200 ergs/mm^2 + $NaAsO_2$	0.4	-1.67 ± 0.75	$-3.15, -0.19$[c]
	0.8	-1.31 ± 0.89	$-3.07, \ 0.45$
	1.2	-2.89 ± 1.14	$-5.15, -0.63$[c]
	1.8	-8.56 ± 0.98	$-10.50, -6.62$[c]

[a]Whole-blood cultures were set from two human subjects for the metal combined with UV light treatment.
[b]Tests of significance were performed for the IF.
[c]IF significant at 95% CI. A positive IF denotes synergy, a negative IF denotes antagonism, and a zero IF denotes additivity.

DISCUSSION

Relatively high doses of Ni(II) increased significantly the SCE frequency compared to untreated control *(13,27)*. We attributed the plateau we observed with increasing concentrations of Ni(II) to the fact that lymphocytes treated with high doses of Ni(II) may have long cell-cycle delays and less severely damaged cells were sampled as M2 metaphases at 68 1/2-h cultures *(29)*.

For the combined treatment of Ni(II) with UV light, the SCE frequency was lower than that expected based on the assumption that the effects of the two damaging agents are additive, with a negative IF *(27)* (Table 1).

Based on the attractive model of SCE formation by Ishii and Bender, the antagonistic interaction of Ni(II) with UV light may be the result of the interference of Ni(II) with the machinery responsible for the formation of SCE *(17,27,30,31)*.

Human lymphocytes treated with nontoxic doses of As(III) induced SCE in a dose-dependent fashion *(13)*, in agreement with previously published results *(19)*. However, combined treatments of As(III) with UV light interacted antagonistically, with an IF ranging from -3.07 to -10.50 (Table 3). Furthermore, at the highest As(III) treatment with UV light, a substantial decrease in the frequency of SCE was observed, suggesting an inhibitory effect in cell proliferation. Antagonistic effects of As(III) have been reported in vitro and in epidemiological studies *(19,26)*. Owing to its clastogenic capabilities, As(III) might inhibit UV light induction of SCE.

The insoluble $PbSO_4$ has been reported to increase significantly the frequency of SCE in cultured hamster cells and in human lymphocytes to induce micronucei (MN) and CAs significantly at doses similar to those tested in our study *(15,16)*. Furthermore this increase was reported to be in a dose-dependent manner, at nontoxic doses of $PbSO_4$. This metal increased the frequency of SCE weakly, but significantly in a dose-dependent manner and reached a plateau at the highest concentration tested *(13)*. This plateau might be attributed to an insoluble precipitate. On addition to the medium of high doses of Pb(II), probably a lead phosphate precipitate was formed *(5)* and phagocytosis did increase the uptake of Pb(II) by cells *(5,32,33)*. This increase in lead uptake could result in a large amount of particulate lead to be taken up by vacuoles or red blood cells, reducing the effect of lead *(33,34)*.

For the combined treatment of Pb(II) with UV light, an almost additive effect was observed. At the highest combined treatment, although the SCE frequency was higher compared to control, it was lower than the other combined treatments *(13)* (Table 2). The lack of a significant antagonistic effect observed for most of the combined treatments is in accord with Ishii and Bender's model of SCE formation *(31)*. Agents that interfere with DNA synthesis may influence the frequencies of UV light-induced SCE *(31)*. Pb(II) has been reported to decrease fidelity and inhibit DNA synthesis *(5,32,33)*, and as a result of these interferences, can increase the SCE induced by UV light. On the other hand, the "bending down" phenomenon observed at the highest combined treatment may be attributed to the fact that Pb(II) decreases protein synthesis and probably histone synthesis, or interferes with unwinding proteins or topoisomerases *(30,31)* and causes a reduction in SCE induced by UV light. Most of lead in blood is found in erythrocytes *(33)*, and red blood cell lysates enhance the frequency of SCE in lymphocytes. Therefore, the idea of a possible toxic effect exerted by relatively high levels of lead as a mechanism of the observed "bending down" phenomenon is eliminated.

The observed differences in the frequency of SCE among experiments is attributed to the type and concentration of metal chelating agents present in the serum among individuals as well as among different batches of serum used for different experiments *(12)*. Moreover, the lack of a linear dose–response may be owing to the inability of ionic metals to enter the cells readily coupled with their relative unrestricted interaction with various cellular ligands *(32)*.

The antagonistic effect of As(III) or Ni(II) combined with mutagens *(17,19,27)* for the induction of SCEs suggests that this assay might have the potential for nonadditive interactions when used to test human exposures to mixtures containing low levels of metals *(26,35)*. Metals affecting certain microsteps in the process of DNA replication or repair (e.g., histones, polymerases, ligases) may have similar antagonistic or enhancing effects.

ACKNOWLEDGMENTS

We thank the Biology Department of St. Francis College for technical assistance.

REFERENCES

1. Costa M, Kraker AJ, Patierno SR. Toxicity and carcinogenicity of essential and nonessential metals. Prog Clin Biochem 1984;1:1–43.
2. Christie NT, Katsifis SP. Nickel carcinogenesis. In: Foulkes EC, ed. Biological Effects of Heavy Metals, vol. II. CRC, Boca Raton, FL, 1990, pp. 95–128.
3. Christie NT, Costa M. In vitro assessment of the toxicity of metal compounds. (II) Effects of Metals on DNA structure and function in intact cells. Biol Trace Element Res 1983;5:55–71.
4. DiPaolo JA, Nelson RL, Casto BC. In vitro neoplastic transformation of SHE cells by lead acetate and its relevance to environmental carcinogenesis. Br J Cancer 1978;38:452–455.
5. Zelikoff JT, Li JH, Hartwig A, Wang XW, Costa M, Rossman TG. Genetic toxicology of lead compounds. Carcinogenesis 1988;9:1727–1732.
6. Pershagen G. The carcinogenicity of arsenic. Environ Health Perspectives 1981;40:93–100.
7. Lee T, Huang R, Jan KY. Sodium arsenite enhances the cytotoxicity, clastogenicity, and 6-thioguanine-resistant mutagenicity of ultraviolet light in Chinese hamster ovary cells. Mutat Res 1985;148:83–89.
8. Wienchke JK, Wrensch MR, Miike R, Petrakis N. Individual susceptibility to induced chromosome damage and its implications for detecting genotoxic exposure in human populations. Cancer Res 1991;51:5266–5269.
9. Hulka BS, Wilcosky T. Biological markers in epidemiologic research. Arch Environ Health 1988;43:83–89.
10. Lambert B, Lindblad A, Holmberg K, Francesconi D. The use of sister chromatid exchange to monitor human populations for exposure to toxicologically harmful agents. In: Wolf S, ed. Sister Chromatid Exchange. John Wiley, New York, 1982, pp. 149–182.
11. Wulf CH. Monitoring of genotoxic exposure of human by the sister chromatid exchange test. Dan Med Bull 1990;37:132–143.
12. Das BC. Factors that influence formation of sister chromatoids exchanges in human blood lymphocytes. CRC Crit Rev Toxicol 1988;19(I):43–86.
13. Sahu RK, Katsifis SP, Kinney PL, Christie NT. Effects of nickel sulfate, lead sulfate, and sodium arsenite alone and with UV light on sister chromatid exchanges in cultured human lymphocytes. J Mol Toxicol 1989;2:129–136.
14. Larramendy ML, Popescu CN, DiPaolo JA. Induction by inorganic metal salts of sister chromatid exchanges and chromosome aberrations in human and Syrian hamster cell strains. Environ Mutagen 1981;3:597–606.
15. Wulf HC. Sister chromatid exchanges in human lymphocytes exposed to nickel and lead. Dan Med Bull 1980;27(1):40–42.
16. Montaldi A, Zentilin L, Zordan M, Bianchi V, Levis AC, Clonfero E, et al. Chromosomal effects of heavy metals (Cd, Cr, Hg, Ni and Pb) on cultured mammalian cells in the presence of nitriloacetic acid. Toxicol Environ Chem 1987;14:183–200.
17. Katsifis SP, Kinney PL, Hosselet S, Burns FJ, Christie NT. Interaction of nickel with mutagens in the induction of sister chromatid exchanges in human lymphocytes. Mutat Res 1996;359:7–15.

18. Wolff S, Bodycote J, Painter RB. Sister chromatid exchanges induced in Chinese hamster cells by UV irradiation of different stages of the cell cycle. The necessity for cells to pass through S. Mutat Res 1974;25:73–81.

19. Wiencke JK, Yager JW. Specificity of arsenite in potentiating cytogenetic damage induced by the DNA crosslinking agent diepoxybutane. Environ Mol Mutagen 1992;19:195–200.

20. Hartwig A, Schlepegrell R, Beyersmann D. Indirect mechanism of lead induced genotoxicity in cultured mammalian cells. Mutat Res 1990;241:75–82.

21. Christie NT. The synergistic interaction of Nickel(II) with DNA damaging agents. Toxicol Environ Chem 1989;22:51–59.

22. Hartwig A, Beyersmann D. Enhancement of UV and chromate mutagenesis by nickel ions in the Chinese hamster HGPRT assay. Toxicol Environ Chem 1987;14:33–42.

23. Casto BC, Meyers J, Di Paolo FA. Enhancement of viral transformation for evaluation of the carcinogenic or mutagenic potential of inorganic lead. Cancer Res 1979;39:193–197.

24. Tanner DC, Lipsky MM. Effect of lead acetate on N-(4-fluoro-4-biphenyl) acetamide-induced renal carcinogenesis in the rat. Carcinogenesis 1984;5:1109–1113.

25. Rossman TG, Meyn SM, Troll W. Effects of arsenite on DNA repair in E. coli. Environ Health Perspectives 1977;19:229–233.

26. Ostrosky-Wegman P, Gonsebatt ME, Montero R, Vega L, Barba H, Espinosa J, et al. Lymphocyte proliferation kinetics and genotoxic findings in a pilot study on individuals chronically exposed to arsenic in Mexico. Mutat Res 1991;250: 477–482.

27 Katsifis SP, Shamy M, Kinney P, Burns FJ. Interaction of nickel with UV-light in the induction of cytogenetic effects in human peripheral lymphocytes. Mutat Res 1998;422(2):331–337..

28. Carrano AV, Natarajan AT. Considerations for populations monitoring using cytogenetic techniques. ICPEMC Publication #14. Mutat Res 1988;204:379–406.

29. Morimoto K, Sato-Mizuno M, Koizumi A. Sister chromatid exchanges and cell cycle kinetics in human lymphocytes cultures exposed to alkylating mutagens: apparent deformity in dose-response relationships. Mutat Res 1985;152:187–196.

30. Dillehay LE, Jacobson-Kram D, Williams JR. DNA topoisomerases models of sister chromatid exchange. Mutat Res 1989;215:15–23.

31. Ishii Y, Bender MA. Effects of inhibitors of DNA synthesis on spontaneous and ultraviolet light-induced sister chromatid exchanges in Chinese hamster cells. Mutat Res 1980;79:19–32.

32. Costa M, Heck JD. Metal Ion carcinogenesis: mechanistic aspects. In: Sigel H, ed. Metal Ions in Biological Systems, vol. 20. Marcel Dekker, New York, 1986, pp. 259–278.

33. Katsifis SP. Metal interaction with physical and chemical agents in the induction of sister chromatid exchanges in human lymphocytes, UMI Dissertation Abstracts Database, Bell & Howell, Ann Arbor MI, PhD Thesis, 1994.

34. Filerman BA, Berliner JA. An in vitro study of the effects of lead on an epithelioid cell line. J Environ Pathol Toxicol 1980;3:491–511.

35. Littorin M, Hogstedt B, Stromback B, Karlsson A, Welinder H, Mitelman S, et al. No cytogenetic effects in lymphocytes of stainless steel welders. Scand J Work Environ Health 1983;9:259–264.

6

The Role of Upper Airway Heat and Water Vapor Exchange in Hygroscopic Aerosol Deposition in the Human Airway

A Deposition Model

Jonathan W. Kaufman, PHD

CONTENTS

INTRODUCTION
METHODS
RESULTS
DISCUSSION
REFERENCES

INTRODUCTION

Physiologically based airway aerosol deposition models provide a quantitative alternative to animal inhalation toxicology testing provided aerosol physicochemical properties are well defined, and sufficient airway anatomical and physiological data are available. Recent airway deposition models deal with the extrathoracic airways (nose, nasopharynx, mouth, oropharynx, and larynx) as a lumped compartment *(1,2)*, or they avoid dealing with the anatomical complexities associated with these airways and use empirical deposition functions *(3)*. These approaches, however, fail to the account for the effect dynamic changes in mucosal blood supply and upper airway geometry (particularly in the oral cavity) can have on regional airway (extrathoracic, tracheobronchial, and pulmonary airways) aerosol deposition. For example, if altering oral cavity

From: *Toxicity Assessment Alternatives: Methods, Issues, Opportunities*
Edited by: H. Salem and S. A. Katz © Humana Press Inc., Totowa, NJ

geometry (moving the tongue) increases oropharyngeal deposition, then pulmonary deposition diminishes because particle numbers decline distal to the upper airway *(4)*.

Extrathoracic particle deposition is especially important for hygroscopic particles. Hydration causes hygroscopic particles to grow and deposit in more proximal airway regions than nonhygroscopic particles of equivalent initial mean mass aerodynamic diameter (MMAD). As a result, fine particles (0.5–2 μm mean mass aerodynamic diameter), which might otherwise pass into tracheobronchial and pulmonary airways, can grow and impact extrathoracic surfaces. This reduces the expected dose in more distal airways by reducing the particle mass reaching these lower airways. Consequently, models that do not adequately account for particle hydration and increased extrathoracic deposition may overestimate pulmonary deposition. This chapter examines how varying extrathoracic heat and water vapor exchange affects hygroscopic particle deposition.

METHODS

A numerical model *(1)* accounting for hygroscopic particle growth was used to predict airway deposition of 0.4 and 1.0 μ MMAD hygroscopic particles. This model estimates regional deposition of mono- or heterodisperse aerosols within the human airway during simulated nasal or oral breathing. Extrathoracic anatomical details were modified in this model, because earlier versions *(1,5)* described the upper airway as a lumped compartment. These modifications conform with anatomical descriptions in the unsteady-state heat and water vapor transport model *(6)* used to generate airway humidity and temperature profiles.

Simulating oral breathing at 16 breaths/min with a 250-mL/s flow rate in 22°C air at 10% RH produced continuous intra- and mass-transfer coefficients that were used as model parameters. In vivo heat and mass-transfer coefficients, h and k_c, were calculated from temperature and airway humidity and temperature profiles. Both in vivo *(7)* and literature *(8)* oral cavity heat humidity data were obtained from a multiple thermocouple probe. This probe simultaneously measured oral cavity wall and airstream temperatures *(7)*. Literature values were obtained from measurements in plastic castings of cadaver upper airways *(8)*. Particle deposition was simulated using the resulting airway humidity and temperature profiles shown in Fig. 1. Both sets of humidity and temperature profiles were input into the deposition model to generate inspiratory regional airway deposition estimates.

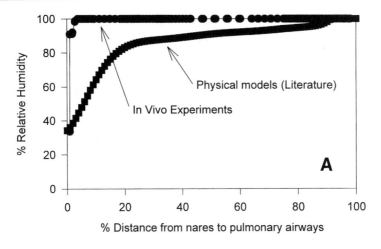

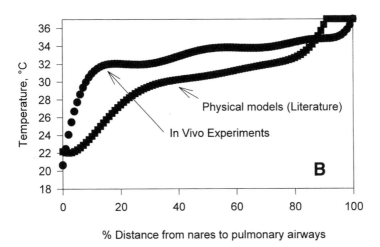

Fig. 1. Simulated human intra-airway (**A**) humidity and (**B**) temperature profiles generated from heat and water vapor exchange data. These profiles provide the basis for simulating human airway hygroscopic particle deposition profiles.

Simulated particles with initial ambient diameters of 0.4 and 1.0 μm MMAD were chosen to model, because hygroscopic particle growth in this size range is particularly sensitive to airway humidity profiles *(7)*. This particle size range corresponds to many inspired airborne toxins, including air pollutants, particles generated by thermal decomposition, most smokes (<3.0 μm), and fly ash *(9)*.

Estimating particle size distribution in a given aerosol is difficult because mechanisms producing the aerosol significantly affect particle sizes. For example, combustion product aerosol particle size distribution is strongly affected by such factors as ignition temperature, latent heat of decomposition, and how a material thermally decomposes *(10)*. In addition, vapor-phase properties and environmental conditions help determine particle size by affecting mechanisms, such as coagulation and condensation, which depend on initial particle composition, charge, hydration, surface area, and shape. These mechanisms can produce wide variation in particle size during combustion. In the present study, a monodisperse aerosol with a particle size geometric standard deviation (σ_g) equal to 1.0 was assumed.

Initial particle composition can be defined in terms of particle ionic strength. Atmospheric water vapor condensing on hygroscopic particle surfaces forms droplets of varying ionic strengths. These droplets grow as a function of ambient relative humidity and particle surface vapor pressure *(11)*. According to Raoult's law *(12)*, surface vapor pressure is a function of solute concentration. Droplets in actual aerosols will have varying solute concentrations depending on initial chemical composition and hydration state. For simplicity, however, inspired particles were modeled as concentrated saline droplets.

RESULTS

Figures 2 and 3 show 0.4- and 1.0-µm MMAD hygroscopic particle intra-airway deposition patterns as a function of human extrathoracic h and k_c obtained from in vivo experiments and physical models of human airways. Predicted extrathoracic and central airway deposition is significantly greater with experimental h and k_c for both 0.4- and 1.0-µm MMAD hygroscopic particles. Extrathoracic deposition of 0.4-µm MMAD particles is predicted to increase by 130%, although deposition of 1.0-µm MMAD particles increases almost 15-fold with experimentally determined h and k_c. Differences in predicted central airway deposition up to about the eighth bronchial generation are equally dramatic. Heat and water vapor exchange rates have little affect on predicted distal airway deposition of 0.4-µm particles. Experimentally determined h and k_c, however, cause predicted 1.0-µm particle deposition to be considerably less than deposition predicted from literature values. Estimated total deposition of 46 and 74% for 0.4- and 1.0-µm MMAD particles, respectively, when using in vivo exchange rates is only 6–10% greater than estimates derived from extrathoracic exchange rates obtained from physical models.

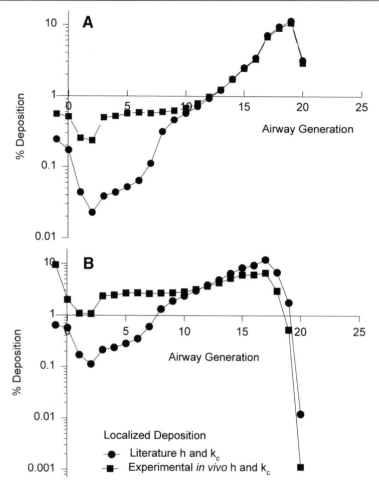

Fig. 2. Predicted localized hygroscopic particle deposition as a function of distance from the pulmonary airways for (**A**) 0.4-μm and (**B**) 1.0-μm MMAD particles. Comparisons are based on simulated humidity and temperature profiles based on in vivo experimental and physical model data.

DISCUSSION

The results demonstrate how extrathoracic heat and water vapor exchange rates affect hygroscopic particle deposition in extrathoracic, central, and distal airways. Values of extrathoracic h and k_c derived from physical models produce simulated deposition profiles in which inspired mass primarily deposits along distal airways. Similar results have been reported in previous work (2,13,14). Using in vivo extrathoracic h and k_c shifts predicted particle deposition to more proximal (extrathoracic

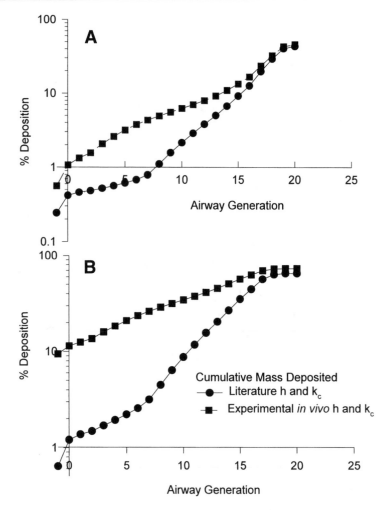

Fig. 3. Predicted cumulative hygroscopic particle deposition as a function of distance from the pulmonary airways for (**A**) 0.4-μm and (**B**) 1.0-μm MMAD particles.

and tracheobronchial) airways. Assuming that this more accurately represents in vivo deposition patterns, inspired 0.4- and 1.0-μm MMAD particles will deposit more along ciliated and squamous epithelium than alveolar endothelium. As a result, predicted physiological responses to inspired pathogenic or pharmaceutical aerosols could change because of possible differences between conducting airway and parenchymal lumenal surface vulnerability and biotransport to submucosal blood vessels.

Distal airway deposition appears dependent on aerosol quantities deposited in extrathoracic airways. For 0.4-μm MMAD hygroscopic particles, extrathoracic deposition is inconsequential (<1% total deposition) for either set (in vivo or physical model) of h and k_c, so most of the aerosol mass remains available for depositing in lower airways. A similar deposition profile with greater total deposition is predicted for 1-μm MMAD particles when simulations are based on physical model extrathoracic h and k_c. Conversely, a large proportion of 1-μm MMAD hygroscopic particles are predicted to impact extrathoracic and central airway surfaces when in vivo h and k_c are used in simulations. This depletes the number and mass of particles available for depositing in lower airways. This relationship between particle size and deposition region conforms to previous findings (2–4,13).

It is noteworthy that using different h and k_c alters the airway region where particles are deposited, but not total deposited mass. Attempting to assess inhalation exposure risk based on total inhaled mass may obscure the risk of localized airway injuries. In a recent human study, Kim et al. (15) observed that dose enhancement occurs at local airway regions, which greatly increases the risk of injury. Therefore, assessing risk of disease or injury only by total inhaled dose appears inadequate. More detailed descriptions of respiratory conditions (flow rates, extrathoracic thermal conditions, inspired airstream physical characteristics) appear necessary for improving risk assessments.

These results call into question the adequacy of current animal inhalation toxicity models. Given that little is known regarding heat and water vapor exchange in rodents, predicting human deposition profiles from rodent deposition studies may be dubious. Proper characterization of key airway and airstream parameters is essential if numerical modeling is to be a reasonable alternative to animal testing. A greater understanding of rodent airway deposition processes is probably necessary before reliable human predictions can be obtained from rodent data. This includes acquiring data on rodent in vivo heat and water vapor exchange and improving existing rodent deposition models. In addition, reliable cross-species correlations also require characterizing human in vivo conditions to a greater extent than currently available data permit.

REFERENCES

1. Persons DD, Hess GD, Muller WJ, Scherer PW. Airway deposition of hygroscopic heterodispersed aerosols: results of a computer calculation. J Appl Physiol 1987;63:1195–1204.
2. Ferron GA, Hornik S. Influence of different humidity profiles on the deposition probability of soluble materials in the human lung. J Aerosol Sci 1984;15:209–211.

3. Martonen TB. Mathematical model for the selective deposition of inhaled pharmaceuticals. J Pharm Sci 1993;82:1191–1199.
4. Kaufman JW, Scherer PW, Yang C-C G. Predicted combustion product deposition in the human airway. Toxicology 1996;115:123–128.
5. Muller WJ, Hess GD, Scherer PW. A model of cigarette smoke particle deposition. Am Ind Hyg Assoc J 1990;51:245–256.
6. Kaufman JW. Human Respiratory Temperature, Water Vapor, and Mucociliary Transport, Ph.D. dissertation. University of Pennsylvania, Philadelphia, 1993.
7. Kaufman JW, Farahmand K, Askew GK. Heat transfer coefficients at the human buccal and tongue surface during quiet breathing. FASEB J 1995;8:A151.
8. Hanna L, Scherer PW. Regional control of local airway heat and water losses. J Appl Physiol 1986;61:624–632.
9. Katz M. City planning, industrial-plant location, and air pollution. In: Magill PL, Holden FR, Ackley C, eds. Air Pollution Handbook. McGraw-Hill, New York, 1956, pp. 2–41.
10. Hilado CJ. Flammability Handbook for Plastics, 3rd ed. Technomic Publishing Westport, CT, 1982, pp. 31–50.
11. Mercer TT. Aerosol Technology in Hazard Evaluation. Academic, New York, 1973, pp. 48–53.
12. Castellan GW. Physical Chemistry, 2nd ed. Addison-Wesley, Reading, MA, 1971, pp. 284–301.
13. Larson TV. The influence of chemical and physical forms of ambient air acids on airway doses. Environ Health Perspectives 1989;79:7–13.
14. Cocks AT, Fernando RP. The growth of sulphate aerosols in the human airways. J Aerosol Sci 1982;13:9–19.
15. Kim CS, Hu SC, DeWitt P, Gerrity TR. Assessment of regional deposition of inhaled particles in human lungs by serial bolus method. J Appl Physiol 1996; 81:2203–2213.

7

Moving Average Interpolation for Malathion LC_{50} Estimation on *Dugesia tigrina*
Comparison with Probit and "One-Point" Methods

R. B. Worobec, PhD

CONTENTS

INTRODUCTION
MATERIALS AND METHODS
RESULTS
DISCUSSION
CONCLUSIONS
REFERENCES

INTRODUCTION

The current political climate as well as moral and ethical consider-ations have had a profound effect on toxicity testing. On the one hand, they have stimulated the development of animal-sparing approaches to dose–response studies and preclinical toxicity testing. On the other hand, they have accelerated the search for alternative assessment models. This confluence of concerns for human health and animal welfare has focused on identification of appropriate animals for a particular health risk, as well as on systems replacing or comple-menting rodent-based experimentation. These alternative options include a variety of bioassays utilizing cell cultures, organ cultures, organelles, whole-embryo cultures, invertebrates, plants, and micro-organisms *(1,2)*.

From: *Toxicity Assessment Alternatives: Methods, Issues, Opportunities*
Edited by: H. Salem and S. A. Katz © Humana Press Inc., Totowa, NJ

Of the various alternative models in use and under development, the free-living freshwater varieties of sexual and asexual planarians—such as the *Dugesia* sp.—are positioned to offer unique advantages in preclinical toxicology in view of their wide spectrum of responses to sundry agents *(3)*. They are the first animals on the phylogenetic scale to exhibit bilateral symmetry, a recognizable central nervous system, encephalization, and a brain to body weight ratio similar to that in rats *(4–7)*. The neurochemical attributes of the planarian central nervous system are in many respects similar to mammals *(8)*, as are their general metabolic characteristics, including detoxifying mechanisms *(9)*. Planarian musculature is similar to that of smooth muscles in higher animals; there is a primitive, but prominent, digestive cavity, while osmoregulation is accomplished by protonephridia *(7,10)*. Planarians are also unique because of their prodigious regenerative capacity, a feature of their developmental biology that has been observed and analyzed for nearly 200 years *(11)*. The latter property has obvious appeal as a model system in studies dealing with cell activation and growth-related phenomena, such as oncogenesis and developmental abnormalities.

Interestingly, in their broad susceptibility to a wide array of toxicants, planarians yield toxicity rankings that are in general analogous to those reported for rodents, although they respond sooner and their relative susceptibility to toxic agents is generally several-fold greater than that of the latter *(7,12)*. On balance, therefore, the biological characteristics of the planarians show them to be very promising objects as in vivo and in vitro models for screening and mechanistic studies of acute, subchronic, and chronic neurotoxicity, genotoxicity, teratogenesis, tumorigenesis, and carcinogenesis *(3,7,9,13–17)*.

The standard approach to determination of the dose or concentration yielding a median effect (i.e., ED_{50}, LD_{50}, IC_{50}, ID_{50}, LC_{50}, and so forth) on the dose–response curve by the probit method requires large numbers of animals for statistical validity and precision *(17–19)*. This fact has led to the development of several alternative methods—and their numerous variations—that require fewer animals and dosage levels, yet offer information meeting the needs of toxicology *(20,21)*. The moving average interpolation (MAI) method is one such alternative development that has been well accepted, and although not a method of curve fitting, has been extended to provide slope estimates *(22,23)*.

This study concentrated on the application of the MAI method to the estimation of malathion median lethal concentration (LC_{50}) vis-a-vis *Dugesia tigrina* for comparison with values obtained by conventional probit analysis and a recently described one-point method *(24)*. Malathion was selected as the test agent since it is a moderately toxic, widely employed pesticide that has been previously tested on planarians *(7,13,14)*, thus providing a broader background for evaluating the applicability of the MAI and one-point approaches to this model.

A MEDLINE search has shown that *Dugesia* sp. are the planarians most often employed in toxicologic studies. For our purposes, *D. tigrina* was selected since it is the most common freshwater planarian encountered in unpolluted streams and ponds in the US *(10)*. *D. tigrina* can thus serve a dual purpose: as an object for preclinical screening of applicable drugs and in monitoring aquatic ecosystem health.

MATERIALS AND METHODS

The study was performed with laboratory cultured asexual *D. tigrina* maintained at $21 \pm 3°C$ in spring water and fed beef liver for 3 h every fifth day. The experiments were carried out under indirect, diffuse daylight in March. The gliding length of animals used in the experiments ranged from 20 to 27 mm. An effort was made to avoid pre- and postfission animals.

Prior to malathion exposure the animals were fasted for 48 h. The malathion preparation employed was an over-the-counter formulation (50% malathion, 50% "inert" ingredients; Ortho Consumer Products, Chevron Chem. Co., San Ramon, CA) adjusted to the appropriate concentration by serial dilution with spring water. The concentrations used were selected to span the LC$_{50}$s previously reported for *Dugesia* sp. exposed to malathion *(7,13,14)*. The experiments were carried out under static conditions, with each worm maintained separately in 5 mL of the highly diluted malathion emulsion.

The 96-h LC$_{50}$ values and their 95% confidence limits (CL) were determined by MAI *(22)*, probit *(25)*, and the newly proposed one-point *(24)* procedures exactly as described.

The MAI study employed 16 flatworms divided equally among the four concentration levels (2, 4, 8, 16 mg/L) of malathion *(22,23)*.

Determination of the 96-h LC$_{50}$ value and its 95% CL by the probit method was accomplished with a program written in BASIC, which includes curve fitting and testing for goodness of fit *(25)*. Six concentrations (1, 2, 4, 8, 16, 32 mg/L) of the malathion formulation were employed, using 10 animals/concentration level, for a total of 60 worms.

Ten planarians were used in the one-point method to gain an estimate of the 96-h LC$_{50}$ and its 95% CL *(24)*, using a 6 mg/L dilution of malathion. Selection of the 6 mg/L concentration for this method was based on the range of LC$_{50}$s previously reported for *D. tigrina* and *D. dorotocephala (7,13,14)*.

In the course of LC_{50} determination the planarians were examined twice a day and signs of behavioral neurotoxicity noted. Animals that appeared to have succumbed to malathion and did not respond to gentle prodding were transferred to fresh spring water and observed for recovery for 2 h.

RESULTS

1. The response of the planarians to malathion consisted of initial agitation, followed by sluggishness and contortion, contraction to a circular form, and eventually dissolution.
2. There were no cases of recovery of planarians that appeared to be dead and failed to respond to gentle tactile stimulation following transfer to fresh spring water.
3. The estimates of the 96-h LC_{50} values and their 95% CLs obtained by the different methods were as follows:

Method	96-h LC_{50} (mg/L)	95% CL (mg/L)
MAI	6.3	4.0–8.6
Probit	5.7	4.9–6.5
One-point	7.2	6.2–8.2

DISCUSSION

Evaluation of the results by the three different approaches yielded overlap in terms of 95% CL ranges among the three sets of results, although barely so when the probit and one-point methods were compared (MAI: 4.0–8.6 mg/L, probit: 4.9–6.5 mg/L, one-point: 6.2–8.2 mg/L.) Nevertheless, considering the myriad of intrinsic and extrinsic factors affecting median dose determinations, the fact that there was overlap of the 95% CL values indicates practical usefulness of all three procedures. In effect, both the MAI procedure and the one-point method have been shown to be valid alternatives for estimating LC_{50} values in this system. The advantage of the 95% CL criterion over determinations of significance of a single LC_{50} value is that it defines a range of parameters that can be accepted or rejected.

The one-point method has recently been successfully applied to LC_{50} determinations in the case of other hydrobionts *(26)*, and appears to be suitable in cases where special emphasis is placed on reduction in the number of animals to be tested and in routine and repetitive screening. Another example of the application of the one-point method would be in isobolographic determination of the nature of drug interactions, an approach that rests on multiple determination of the median effective dose of a drug combination *(27)*. In passing, it should be mentioned that the MAI approach can also be used with as few as two dosage levels *(28)*.

The respective number of animals required in the MAI, one-point, and probit procedures were 16, 10, and 60 planarians. Determination of the median effect concentrations by the classical probit methodology depends on a relatively large number of animals for statistical validity and precision, which is a definite disadvantage if expensive or large animals are involved *(19)*. In the case of planarians, however, this need not be a concern since they can be raised and maintained easily and inexpensively in populations of tens of thousands. However, in most cases—and in special cases where observations have to be performed on individual specimens—economy of animals and time makes sense in screening. Finally, the selection of an over-the-counter malathion product was based on the assumption that it is precisely this type of formulation that is involved in ordinary human exposure and pollution of the aquatic milieu, thereby posing a potential health hazard in the real world *(29,30)*.

As already noted, planarians offer many interesting features that make them suitable for toxicity assessment as a model system complementary to higher animals. Their susceptibility to the adverse developmental effects of thalidomide *(1,16)* and neurotoxic manifestations of methyl-mercury *(1,7)* does conjure up the human tragedies of phocomelia and Minamata disease as the respective consequences of inadequate pre-clinical testing and indifference to environmental pollution.

Considering the information available on the planarians, their biology, responsiveness to toxic agents, and natural habitat, it appears that they should be further developed as sentinel organisms for monitoring freshwater ecosystems and in preliminary human safety evaluation. They are inexpensive, readily available, and are easy to raise, maintain, and manipulate.

CONCLUSIONS

- In the *D. tigrina*-malathion system moving average interpolation and the one-point method have been validated as giving 96-h LC$_{50}$ values comparable to those obtained with the classical probit approach in terms of 95% CL overlap. However, the former two methods required far fewer animals than did the probit procedure.
- The results provided by the moving average method are much closer to those given by the benchmark probit approach than the results obtained with the one-point method in this system and, in addition, the moving average method can also be used to estimate the slope.
- Planarians constitute a valid, inexpensive, and easily managed complementary or even alternative model in certain preclinical safety testing situations. They are also an obvious candidate as sentinel organisms in monitoring the health of freshwater aquatic ecosystems.

REFERENCES

1. Goss LB, Sabourin TD. Utilization of alternative species for toxicity testing: an overview. J Appl Tox 1985;5:193–219.
2. Salem H, ed., Animal Test Alternatives: Refinement, Reduction, Replacement. Marcel Dekker, New York, 1995.
3. Best JB, Morita M. Toxicology of planarians. Hydrobiologia 1991;227:375–383.
4. Palladini G, Margotta V, Carolei A, Chiarini F, Del Piano M, Lauro GM, et al. The cerebrum of *Dugesia gonocephala* s.1. Platyhelminthes, Turbellaria, Tricladida. Morphological and functional observations. J Hirnforsch 1983;24:165–172.
5. Sarnat HB, Netsky MG. The brain of the planarian as the ancestor of the human brain. Can J Neurol Sci 1985;12:296–302.
6. Best JB, Abelein M, Kreutzer E, Pigon A. Cephalic mechanisms for social control of fissioning in planarians: III. Central nervous system centers of facilitation and inhibition. J Comp Physiol Psychol 1975;89:923–932.
7. Best JB. Transphyletic animal similarities and predictive toxicology. In: van der Merve A, ed., Old and New Questions in Physics, Cosmology, Philosophy, and Theoretical Biology, Essays in Honor of Wolfgang Yourgrau. Plenum, New York, 1983, pp. 549–591.
8. Reuter M, Gustafson MKS. The flatworm nervous system: pattern and phylogeny. Experientia Suppl (Basel) 1995;72:25–59.
9. Schaeffer DJ. Planarians as a model system for *in vivo* teratogenesis studies. Qual Assess: Good Pract, Regul Law 1993;2:265–318.
10. Hyman LH. The Invertebrates, vol. II, Platyhelminthes and Rhynchocoela; The Acoelomate Bilateralia. McGraw-Hill, New York, 1951, p. 533.
11. Brondsted HV. Planarian regeneration. Biol Rev 1955;30:65–126.
12. Worobec RB. Rapid assessment of pesticide toxicity on planaria [abstract]. In: Chemical Mixtures and Quantitative Risk Assessment, 2nd Annual Symposium, Nov. 7–10, 1994, Raleigh, NC, Health Effects Research Laboratory, US EPA, Research Triangle Park, NC, 1994.
13. Villar D, Li M-H, Schaeffer DJ. Toxicity of organophosphorus Pesticides to *Dugesia dorotocephala*. Bull Environ Contam Toxicol 1993;51:80–87.
14. Villar D, Gonzales M, Gualda MJ, Schaeffer DJ. Effects of organophosphorus insecticides on Dugesia tigrina: Cholinesterase activity and head regeneration. Bull Environ Contam Toxicol 1993;52:319–324.
15. Schaeffer DJ. Planarians as a model system for *in vivo* tumorigenesis studies. Ecotoxicol Environ Safety 1993;25:1–18.
16. Best JB, Morita M. Planarians as a model system for *in vitro* teratogenesis studies. Teratogenesis Carcinog Mutagen 1982;2:277–291.
17. Schaeffer DJ, Tehseen WM, Johnson LR, McLaughlin GL, Hassan AS, Reynolds HA, et al. Cocarcinogenesis between cadmium and Arochlor 1254 in planarians is enhanced by inhibition of glutathione synthesis. Qual Assess: Good Pract, Regul Law 1991;1:31–41.
18. Trevan JW. The error of determination of toxicity. Proc R Soc (Lond) Ser B 1927;101:483–514.
19. Litchfield JT, Wilcoxon F. A simplified method of evaluation dose effect experiments. J Pharmacol Exp Ther 1949;96:99–113.
20. Paumgartten FJR, Presgrave OAF, Menezes MAC, Fingola FF, Freitas JC, Carvalho RR, et al. Comparison of five methods for the determination of lethal dose in acute toxicity studies. Brazil J Med Biol Res 1989;22:987–991.

21. Depass LR. Alternative approaches in median lethality (LD$_{50}$) and acute toxicity testing. Toxicol Lett 1989;49:159–170.

22. Weil CS. Tables for convenient calculation of median-effective dose (LD$_{50}$ or ED$_{50}$) and instructions in their use. Biometrics 1952;8:249–263.

23. Weil CS. Economical LD$_{50}$ and slope determinations. Drug Chem Toxicol 1983;6:595–603.

24. Frumin GT. Rapid method for determination of effective and lethal doses (concentrations). Khim-Farmatsevt Zh 1991;25:15–18 [in Russian].

25. Lieberman HR. Estimating LD$_{50}$ using the probit technique: a BASIC computer program. Drug Chem Toxicol 1983;6:111–116.

26. Frumin GT, Chuiko GM, Pavlov DF, Menzykova OV. New rapid method to evaluate the median effect concentrations of xenobiotics in hydrobionts. Bull Env Contam Toxicol 1992;49:361–367.

27. Gessner PK. Isobolographic analysis of interactions: an update on applications and utility. Toxicology 1995;105:161–179.

28. Depass LR, Myers RC, Weaver EV, Weil CS. An assessment of the importance of number of dosage levels, number of animals per dosage level, sex and method of LD$_{50}$ and slope calculation in acute toxicity studies. Alt Methods Toxicol 1984;2:140–153.

29. Desi G, Dura L, Gonczi Z, Kneffel Z, Strohmayer A, Szabo Z. Toxicity of malathion to mammals, aquatic organisms and tissue culture cells. Arch Env Contam Toxicol 1975/76;3:410–425.

30. Flessel P, Quintana PJE, Hooper K. Genetic toxicity of malathion: a review. Env Mol Mutag 1993;22:7–17.

8 Physiological Modeling of Benzo(a)pyrene Pharmacokinetics in the Rat

David Moir, PHD

CONTENTS

INTRODUCTION

In spite of the title of this chapter being relatively specific, the bulk of it will be of a more general nature in an attempt to describe the current state of physiologically based pharmacokinetic (PBPK) modeling and where efforts will likely be directed in the future. Some of the newer approaches to parameter estimation will then be used in the specific case of modeling the pharmacokinetics of benzo(a)pyrene (B[a]P) in the rat.

Modeling the disposition of chemicals based on the physiology of the exposed organism has a longer history than is often realized. Figure 1 shows a time line with some of the more significant developments in the past 70 years. The first person to attempt to use the physiology of the animal as a determinant in modeling the disposition of a chemical was Haggard *(1)* in 1924, when he considered the inhalation of diethyl ether. More than a decade later, Teorell *(2)* described, from a physiological point of view, the determinants of drug disposition, but was unable to solve the resultant equations. In the early 1950s, Kety *(3)* described the biological system as an array of parallel physiological compartments interconnected by the systemic circulation, a representation that is still

From: *Toxicity Assessment Alternatives: Methods, Issues, Opportunities*
Edited by: H. Salem and S. A. Katz © Humana Press Inc., Totowa, NJ

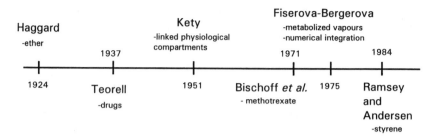

Fig. 1. Time line showing some of the significant contributions in the development of PBPK modeling.

in use today. In 1971, Bischoff et al. *(4)* successfully modeled the disposition of several doses of methotrexate in rats. Fiserova-Bergerova *(5)* modeled inhaled vapors and used numerical integration to "solve" the differential equations. In 1984, Ramsey and Andersen *(6a)* published their landmark PBPK model on the inhalation of styrene in the rat and human. The basic structure of this model is still in use today, and that paper clearly demonstrated that PBPK modeling can be useful in hazard identification and risk assessment.

Model Structure

PBPK models have the same basic structure that Kety *(3)* initially described: a series of parallel compartments linked by blood (Fig. 2). The number of compartments will depend on the chemical and its disposition, but in general, any compartment that metabolizes the chemical will be included, as will any compartment that sequesters or binds the chemical. There will also be a compartment to allow for the introduction of the chemical, as for example, lung in the case of an inhaled substance, and if not already included, the target organ of toxic substances will also form part of the model. The rest of the animal is often described by two lumped compartments, one consisting of richly perfused tissues, and the other of poorly perfused tissues. All of these compartments are connected by blood flow in a physiologically relevant fashion, with the total cardiac output of venous blood entering the lung and arterial blood leaving the lung to be apportioned among the various compartments according to their relative blood flows.

Model Description

The majority of PBPK models to date have been for volatile organics *(6b)*. This is owing in part to the commercial and industrial importance of volatile organics; this widespread use leads to occupational expo-

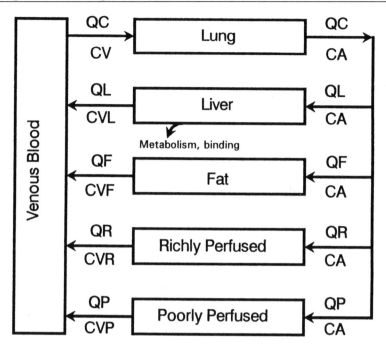

Fig. 2. Conceptual representation of a general PBPK model where the Qs represent blood flow rates, the Cs are concentrations in arterial or venous blood and in venous blood leaving the tissues.

sure of workers and allows the generation of excellent estimates of average daily exposure or lifetime exposures, which are critical to epidemiological studies. The continuing requirement for better risk assessments of important chemicals and the ability of PBPK models to extrapolate from dose to dose, route to route, and species to species have combined to focus the attention of those active in PBPK modeling on volatile organics. PBPK models of volatiles usually describe tissues with a flow limitation (Fig. 3), meaning that the amount of chemical available to a tissue is dependent on the rate of blood flow to it. An assumption is made that the compartment is homogenous and well mixed, and the rate of change of the amount of a chemical in the tissue can be described by a single equation (Eq. 1):

$$(dAT/dt) = QT\,(CA - CVT) \tag{1}$$

where AT is the amount in mg of chemical in tissue, QT is the blood flow in L/h to the tissue, CA is the concentration of chemical in arterial blood, and CVT is the concentration of chemical in venous blood leaving the tissue. The concentration of venous blood leaving the tissue is related to

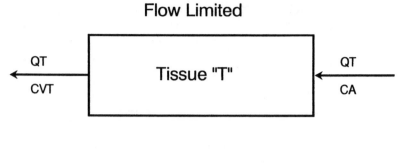

$$\frac{dAT}{dt} = VT \times \frac{dCT}{dt} = QT(CA\text{-}CVT)$$

$$CVT = \frac{CT}{PC}$$

Fig. 3. The rate of change in the amount of chemical in a flow-limited tissue is equal to the concentration in arterial blood (CA) less the concentration in venous blood leaving the tissue (CVT) times the blood flow to the tissue (QT).

the concentration in the tissue *(CT)* by the tissue to blood partition coefficient *(PC)* in the following fashion (Eq. 2):

$$CVT = (CT/PC) \tag{2}$$

For nonvolatiles, especially of higher molecular weight, diffusion can be the rate-limiting step. To model the rate of change in tissues in this case, a separate tissue blood subcompartment must be created. The rate of change of the amount of chemical in the tissue is equal to the product of the permeation area crossproduct PA_t and the net flux from the tissue blood (Eq. 3).

$$(dAT/dt) = PA_t \left[CVT - (CT/PC) \right] \tag{3}$$

The rate of change in the tissue blood subcompartment equals the net retention from blood flow plus the net flux from the tissue proper (Eq. 4):

$$(dAT_B/dt) = QT (CA - CVT) + PA_t \left[(CT/PC) - CVT \right] \tag{4}$$

where AT_B is the amount of chemical in the tissue blood.

Parameter Estimation

The appeal of pharmacokinetic modeling comes from the possibility of estimating tissue dose in different species and under different exposure conditions. A model that describes the behavior of a chemical can be related to the biological response of the organism to that chemical.

Coupled with the possibility for extrapolation, PBPK modeling is especially attractive in risk-assessment applications.

There are three types of parameters that are required for the construction of these types of models: physiological, physicochemical, and biochemical. Physiological parameters relate to the animal and are often scaled to body weight. Examples of these are cardiac output, tissue blood flow rates, tissue volumes and weights, ventilation rates, and so forth. In general, these parameters are readily available in the literature for a number of species (e.g., 7). Examples of physicochemical parameters that are required are tissue to blood PCs and diffusion coefficients. These parameters must be estimated. For volatile organics, tissue to blood PCs are almost always estimated by the vial equilibration technique of Sato and Nakajima (8) as modified by Gargas et al. (9). This reliable technique estimates the tissue to air and blood to air PCs by head space analysis, and the quotient of these provides an estimate of the tissue to blood PC. No such reliable method for nonvolatiles exists, although there are a number of recent papers that offer alternatives.

The earliest method for nonvolatile tissue to blood PC estimations involved in vivo constant infusion (10) in which the animal was infused until a pseudo-steady state was attained. Organ and plasma residue levels allowed the estimation of the PCs, but the method suffered from the fact that the system was not truly at steady state. The remainder of the methods are in vitro techniques. The equilibrium dialysis method (11) involves dialyzing tissue homogenate or blood against a buffered solution of the radiolabeled chemical at several different concentrations. The drawbacks to this method are the requirement for radiolabeled material and the length of time required for adipose tissue to reach equilibrium. Jepson et al. (12) recently published a method that may have general applicability for nonvolatiles. Tissue or blood was incubated with the chemical of interest and then centrifuged. A portion of the supernatant was filtered under pressure through a membrane with a mol-wt cutoff of 10,000. The filtrate was then extracted and analyzed in a chemical-specific fashion. There has been a report of some analyte binding to the plastic of the filtration device (13), but this will vary with the chemical. Murphy et al. (14) have described a PC-determination method that is analogous to Gargas' (9) vial equilibration method. This uses a solvent, in this case propylene carbonate, as a surrogate for the air in the headspace technique. The PCs between blood and propylene carbonate and tissue homogenates and propylene carbonate were determined for 2,3,7,8-tetrachlorodioxin and for estradiol, and gave good agreement with previously published PCs. There are two features of this method that will likely limit its applicability: as used here, the method requires radiolabeled material, and the selection of the "surrogate" solvent is critical. Not only must the solvent be immiscible with saline and the tissue homogenates and blood, but it must also solubilize the test chemical to the slightest extent possible to allow partitioning into the tissues.

Poulin and Krishnan *(15)* have developed a biologically based algorithm for PC estimation. This method requires the octanol:water PC, which is often available in the literature, along with lipid content and type in the tissues of interest. The equation for partitioning into tissues (P_t) is:

$$P_t = (K_{O/W} \times F_{nt}) + (1 \times F_{wt}) + (K_{O/W} \times 0.3 \times F_{pt}) + (1 \times 0.7 \times F_{pt}) \quad (5)$$

where $K_{O/W}$ is the octanol:water PC, and F is the fraction of tissue weight of neutral lipids (F_{nt}), water in tissue (F_{wt}), and phospholipids (F_{pt}). This was extrapolated to rat erythrocyte and plasma:

$$P_e = (K_{O/W} \times F_{\neq}) + (1 \times F_{we}) + (K_{O/W} \times 0.3 \times F_{pe}) + (1 \times 0.7 \times F_{pe}) \quad (6)$$

$$P_p = (K_{O/W} \times F_{np}) + (1 \times F_{wp}) + (K_{O/W} \times 0.3 \times F_{pp}) + (1 \times 0.7 \times F_{pp}) \quad (7)$$

where the subscript "e" refers to erythrocytes and the subscript "p" refers to plasma. The relative contribution of erythrocyte and plasma to the partitioning was based on the composition of rat blood to give the final equation:

$$P_{tb} = [P_t/(0.37 \times P_e) + (0.63 \times P_p)] \quad (8)$$

Good agreement was obtained when comparing PCs estimated using the algorithm with those obtained experimentally, generally using the vial equilibration method. The availability of tissue to blood PCs for a large number of volatile chemicals has allowed the validation of this method, which suggests that it could become the accepted method for the estimation of PCs for nonvolatile chemicals. The last method that has been applied to nonvolatiles is that of optimization, in which all parameters are fixed save the PCs. These are then varied within limits, the fit of the simulation to data is assessed in some way, and the "best" set of PCs is determined. An example of this can be found in the work of Andersen et al. *(16)* in their model on dioxin and receptors. They used previously published PCs as starting points, and then optimized to fit their data. This type of approach has the drawback of varying multiple parameters, which can potentially give any number of possible solutions.

The biochemical constants required for the construction of PBPK models generally include metabolism constants to describe first-order (K_f) or saturable (K_m, V_{max}) biotransformation processes, and may also require constants to describe absorption or binding. Metabolism constants have been estimated using in vivo and in vitro techniques along with extrapolation methods. The in vivo techniques have been most often used with volatile organics and include some truly innovative methods, such as closed-chamber gas uptake *(17,18)* and the exhaled breath analysis method *(19).* In the closed-chamber method, animals are exposed to a recirculated atmosphere containing a volatile organic. The decline in concentration of this chemical in chamber air is owing to uptake and metabolism by these animals. The exhaled breath analysis method uses an animal that has been exposed to a chemical, and then is placed in a flowthrough chamber equipped with a sampling port for chromatographic analysis. In this case, any chemical in the chamber air has been exhaled by the animal and is a reflection of the blood levels of this chemical. In both of the above methods, the data points are fitted using a PBPK model by optimizing the metabolic constants. Another in vivo method has been applied to estimate the metabolic constants for dibromomethane biotransformation. This stable metabolite technique can be used only in the case of metabolites that are not further transformed and ideally are created in the first step of metabolism. The only example of this has been the production of bromide ion from dibromomethane as described by Gargas et al. *(20).*

There are numerous in vitro techniques for kinetic constant determination, all of which apply to liver, but some can also be used with lung or kidney, or any organ that metabolizes the chemical. These methods include the use of perfused whole organ, tissue slices, S-9 fractions, microsomes, cultured hepatocytes, and cytosols. Each method has advantages and disadvantages. Although rate constants have been determined for numerous chemicals using in vitro methods, only a few of these constants have been used directly in PBPK models *(21).* This is because there is often not a good correlation between in vitro and in vivo studies. Bisgaard and Lam *(22)* have considered the qualitative differences in the production of metabolites from 1,3-diaminobenzene using perfused rat liver, hepatocytes, microsomes, and the whole rat. In this study, only the hepatocytes produced a metabolite profile consistent with that found in the whole animal. Some in vitro methods are better than others, and exactly which one is most suitable will depend on the chemical and the manner in which it is metabolized. The great appeal of PBPK models comes from their ability to extrapolate, either dose to dose, route to route, or species to species. In the case of application to risk assessment, these models must estimate the fate of the chemical in humans, and very often the metabolic parameters must be estimated in some fashion. This has generally been done by extrapolation in one of several ways. A parallelogram approach was developed by Reitz et al. *(23)* to estimate human in vivo rate constants for use in the risk assessment of dichloromethane, and this approach is still being used today

(24,25). To apply this method, animal in vivo and in vitro data are required, as are human in vitro data. An assumption is made that the ratio of activity in vivo to in vitro is the same across species. The activity ratio in rat is applied to in vitro activity in humans to give an estimate of activity in vivo in human. A different approach is the extrapolation from in vivo animal data to in vivo human *(24,26)*. This requires in vivo data on the chemical of interest and on similar chemical(s) in the test species, as well as in vivo data on that similar chemical(s) in humans. The rate constant in humans is estimated by multiplying the rate constant in the test species by the ratio of rates, human to test species, on the similar chemical(s). Reitz et al. *(24)* applied both of the above techniques to the estimation of human rate constants for perchloroethylene and arrived at a human V_{max} (mg/h) of 25.4 using the extrapolation approach and 41.5 using the parallelogram approach.

Benzo(a)pyrene Pharmacokinetics

We have applied some of the above techniques in the construction of a PBPK model to describe the pharmacokinetics of B(a)P in the rat. Although this chemical has been extensively studied, there has been little attention paid to its pharmacokinetics. In 1959, Kotin et al. *(27)* described some blood concentration–time-course data for rats dosed at 55 µg/kg. Schlede et al. *(28)* provided some tissue concentration–time-course data, notably for liver and adipose, at about the same dosage. Weirsma and Roth *(29)* considered the effect of pretreatment of rats with 3-methylcholanthrene on the kinetics of removal of B(a)P from blood. In 1990, Roth and Vinegar *(30)* constructed a PBPK model for B(a)P in the rat using the values from the earlier study by Schlede et al. *(28)*. Because of the limited time-course data available, we decided to conduct a thorough pharmacokinetic study on B(a)P. Briefly, this study employed 3 dose levels and 15 sampling intervals ranging from 5 min to 32 h. ^{14}C-labeled B(a)P was injected into male rats at 2, 6, or 15 mg/kg body wt. Tissues and blood were analyzed for total ^{14}C-content and for B(a)P itself by high-performance liquid chromatography (HPLC). The extraction method for nonadipose tissue employed dichloromethane and cleanup with Florisil *(31)*. Adipose tissue was extracted using a method that capitalized on the differential partitioning of B(a)P and lipids in hexane and dimethyl sulfonide (DMSO) *(32)*. This data set, specifically the 15 mg/kg group, was used as a calibration set in the construction of the PBPK model.

The model consists of six compartments: liver, adipose, lung, richly perfused tissue group, poorly perfused tissue group, and venous blood. The physiological parameters were from Arms and Travis *(7)*, except

Table 1
Tissue to Blood PCs as Determined
by Equilibrium Dialysis

Tissue	PC
Liver	2.31
Adipose	7.78 (438)[a]
Richly perfused	1.60
Poorly perfused	0.69
Lung	1.78

[a]From algorithm of Poulin and Krishnan (15).

cardiac output was 0.233 L/min/kg (33), and fraction of body weight as fat tissue was 0.09 kg/kg body wt (6a). The required tissue to blood PCs were estimated by the equilibrium dialysis method. Tissue homogenates and blood were dialyzed against buffered solutions of 5 different concentrations of radiolabeled B(a)P, ranging from 0.05 to 0.6 mM. The tissue to buffer PCs were divided by the blood to buffer PCs to give the tissue to blood PCs. The richly perfused PCs were estimated by combining PCs for kidney, brain, and heart, according to their relative blood flows. The PC for poorly perfused tissue group was taken to be the same as muscle to blood (see Table 1).

All simulations were run using the program ScOP (Simulation Resources Inc., Berrien Springs, MI). Initial simulations using the above PCs indicated that the PC for adipose tissue was substantially lower than necessary to fit the data. Understanding that adipose tissue is slow to reach equilibrium in the tissue dialysis experiments prompted the use of the algorithm approach of Poulin and Krishnan (15) to generate an estimate for adipose PC, while still using the dialysis PCs for the remaining tissues. The biochemical constants were taken from the literature (29). Hepatic V_{max} as determined by a microsomal preparation was 0.244 mg/kg/min, and the Michaelis constant K_m was 1.386 mg/L. Pulmonary constants were a V_{max} of 0.0001 mg/kg/min and K_m of 0.055 mg/L.

From the outset, there was an expectation that some tissues would require a diffusion limitation. This could be determined by considering the distribution phase of the kinetic profile, i.e., immediately after injection, in the absence of metabolism. If the simulation provided numbers that were much greater than the data points, then a diffusion limitation must be included. In this model, this limitation is accomplished by use of a fractional diffusion parameter, which serves essentially to limit blood flow from the tissue blood subcompartment to the tissue itself. If this parameter is set to 1.0, there is no diffusion, and the tissue is considered to be flow-

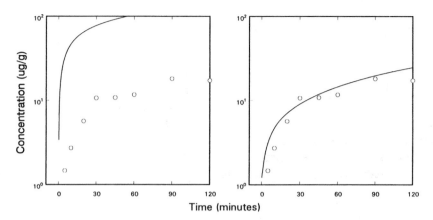

Fig. 4. Model simulations (lines) of B(a)P concentrations in adipose tissue over time with (right graph) and without (left graph) diffusion limitation plotted with data points (open circles) from the pharmacokinetic study. No metabolism is active in the model ($V_{max} = 0$).

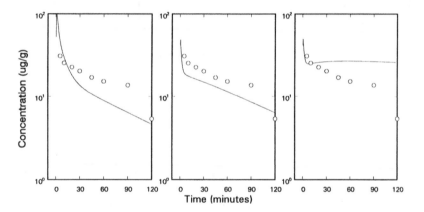

Fig. 5. Model simulations (lines) of B(a)P concentrations in richly perfused tissue over time with (middle graph) and without diffusion limitation. The right graph shows the simulation with both richly perfused and adipose tissue with diffusion limitations. The data points (open circles) are from kidney.

limited. Each tissue was checked, and adipose (Fig. 4) and the richly perfused tissue group (Fig. 5) were found to require the diffusion limitation.

With these diffusion parameters in the model, the metabolism was turned back on, and as shown in Fig. 6, all simulations underestimated the experimental values in all tissues. It was apparent that the hepatic V_{max} of 0.244 mg/min/kg was an inappropriate value. This value was estimated using a microsomal enzyme preparation, which often does not

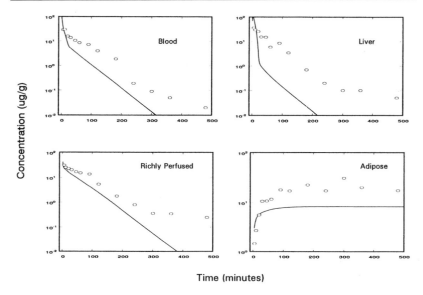

Time (minutes)

Fig. 6. Model simulations (lines) of B(a)P concentrations in four tissue groups over time with V_{max} = 0.244 mg/min/kg.

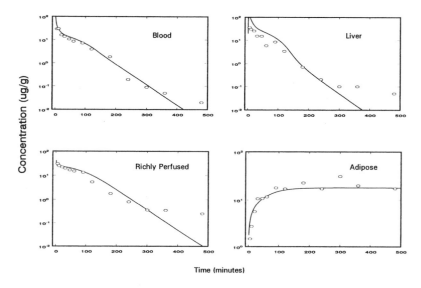

Time (minutes)

Fig. 7. Model simulations (lines) of B(a)P concentrations in four tissue groups over time with V_{max} = 0.06 mg/min/kg.

extrapolate well from in vitro to in vivo. Consequently, the V_{max} was optimized interactively to a value of 0.06 mg/min/kg, and the simulations for the various tissues at a dose level of 15 mg/kg are shown in Fig. 7.

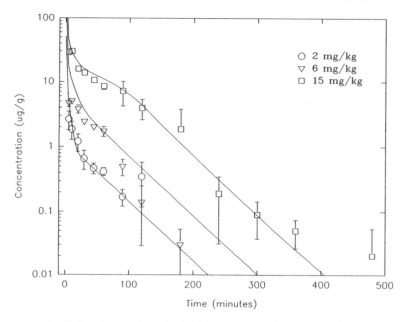

Fig. 8. Model simulations (lines) of B(a)P concentrations in blood over time at three concentrations: 2, 6, and 15 mg/kg body wt.

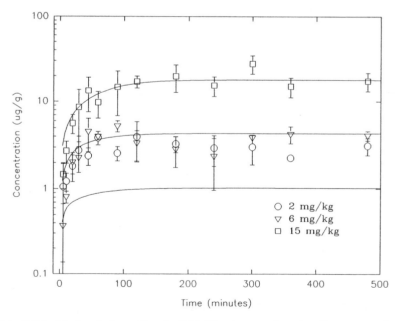

Fig. 9. Model simulations (lines) of B(a)P concentrations in adipose over time at three concentrations: 2, 6, and 15 mg/kg body wt.

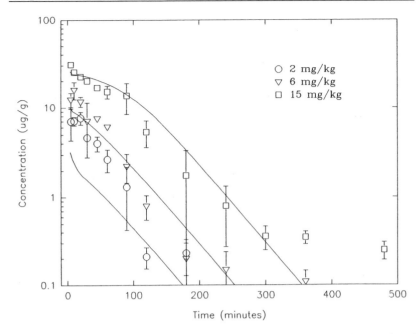

Fig. 10. Model simulations (lines) of B(a)P concentrations in richly perfused tissue over time at three concentrations: 2, 6, and 15 mg/kg body wt, as compared to data points from kidney.

To validate the model, it is necessary to check it against various data sets. Figures 8–11 show the simulations and experimental data points for the three dose levels of 2, 6, and 15 mg/kg in the various tissue groups. The data points in the richly perfused graph (Fig. 10) are from kidney. In general, there is good agreement between the simulations and the experimental data, with two notable exceptions. The fit to the liver data is the poorest of any of the tissues, likely because of the well-known property of B(a)P to bind to receptors. Inclusion of a binding term, similar to that used by Travis and Bowers *(34)*, will likely improve the fit. The second poor fit is to the 2 mg/kg data for adipose. It is believed that this is a function of the analytical method, and that the experimental values are overestimating the true values.

The only other time-course data available are from Schlede et al. *(28),* and the simulations to these data are shown in Fig. 12. Good fit is obtained for blood and adipose, but again the fit is poor for the liver. These data from Schlede et al. were obtained at a dose level of 56 µg/kg body wt, as compared to up to 15 mg/kg in the present study, so the model holds equally well over a very large exposure range. Table 2 summarizes the origin of parameters to be found in the Roth and Vinegar *(30)* model

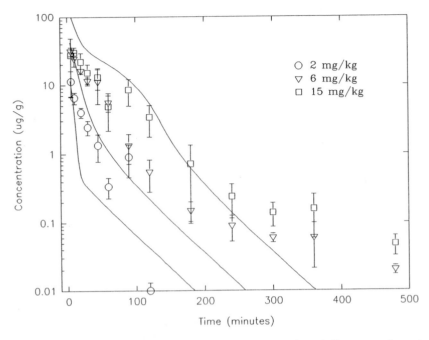

Fig. 11. Model simulations (lines) of B(a)P concentrations in liver over time at three concentrations: 2, 6, and 15 mg/kg body wt.

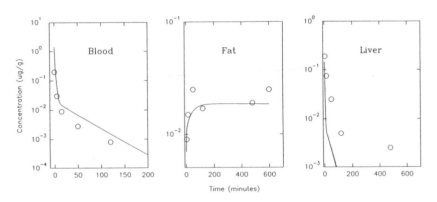

Fig. 12. Model simulations (lines) of B(a)P concentrations in blood, fat, and liver plotted against the values of Schlede et al. *(28)* at 56 μg/kg.

and the model presented here. Generally, the more parameters fitted by optimization, the less confidence that can be placed in the model.

In summary, this chapter has attempted to describe some of the tools available to modelers and risk assessors, especially with regard to

Table 2
Origin of Parameters for B(a)P PBPK Models

Parameter	Roth and Vinegar (30)	This model
Physiological	Fixed	Fixed
V_{max}	In vitro	Fitted
K_m	In vitro	In vitro
PCs	Fitted	In vitro; algorithm
Diffusion parameters	—	Fitted

nonvolatile compounds. This field is likely to see a concentration of effort toward improving in vitro to in vivo correlations and interspecies extrapolations.

ACKNOWLEDGMENTS

It is a pleasure to acknowledge the contributions of my collaborators: K. Krishnan, Université de Montréal for modeling guidance; F. C. P. Law, Simon Fraser University, for the partition coefficients for B(a)P; Ih Chu for pharmacokinetic guidance; and André Viau for excellent technical assistance on the tissue analyses.

REFERENCES

1. Haggard HW. The absorption, distribution and elimination of ethyl ether. Analysis of the mechanism of the absorption and elimination of such a gas or vapor as ethyl ether. J Biol Chem 1924;59:753–770.
2. Teorell T. Kinetics of distribution of substances administered to the body. I. The extravascular modes of administration. Arch Int Pharmacodyn 1937;57:205–225.
3. Kety SS. The theory and application of the exchange of inert gas at the lungs. Pharmacol Rev 1951;3:1–41.
4. Bischoff KB, Dedrick RL, Zakharo DS, Longstreth JA. Methotrexate pharmacokinetics. J Pharm Sci 1971;60:1128–1133.
5. Fiserova-Bergerova V. Mathematical modeling of inhalation exposure. J Combust Toxicol 1975;32:201–210.
6a. Ramsey JC, Andersen ME. A physiologically-based description of the inhalation pharmacokinetics of styrene in rats and humans. Toxicol Appl Pharmacol 1984;73:159–175.
6b. Krishnan K, Andersen ME. Physiologically based pharmacokinetic modeling in toxicology. In: Hayes AW, ed. Principles and Methods of Toxicology. Raven, New York, 1994, pp. 149–188.
7. Arms AD, Travis CC. Reference physiological parameters in pharmacokinetic modeling. Office of Health and Environmental Assessment, US EPA, Washington, DC, NTIS PB88-196019, 1988.
8. Sato A, Nakajima T. Partition coefficients of some aromatic hydrocarbons and ketones in water, blood and oil. Br J Ind Med 1979;36:231–234.

9. Gargas ML, Burgess RJ, Voisard DE, Cason GH, Andersen ME. Partition coefficients of low-molecular-weight volatile chemicals in various liquids and tissues. Toxicol Appl Pharmacol 1989;98:87–99.

10. Chen HSG, Gross JF. Estimation of tissue to plasma partition coefficients used in physiological pharmacokinetic models. J Pharmacokinet Biopharm 1979;7:117–125.

11. Lin J, Sugiyama Y, Awazu S, Hanano M. *In vitro* and *in vivo* evaluation of the tissue-to-blood partition coefficient for physiological pharmacokinetic models. J Pharmacokinet Biopharmacol 1982;10:637–647.

12. Jepson GW, Hoover DK, Black RK, McCafferty JD, Mahle DA, Gearhart JM. A partition coefficient determination method for nonvolatile chemicals in biological tissues. Fundam Appl Toxicol 1994;22:519–524.

13. Knaak JB, Albayati MA, Raabe OG. Development of partition coefficients, V_{max} and K_m values, and allometric relationships. Toxicol Lett 1995;79:87–98.

14. Murphy JE, Janszen DB, Gargas ML. An *in vitro* method for determination of tissue partition coefficients of non-volatile chemicals such as 2,3,7,8-tetrachlorodibenzo-*p*-dioxin and estradiol. J Appl Toxicol 1995;15:147–152.

15. Poulin P, Krishnan K. An algorithm for predicting tissue:blood partition coefficients of organic chemicals from n-octanol:water partition coefficient data. J Toxicol Environ Health 1995;46:117–129.

16. Andersen ME, Mills JJ, Gargas ML, Kedderis L, Birnbaum LS, Neubert D, et al. Modeling receptor-mediated processes with dioxin: implications for pharmacokinetics and risk assessment. Risk Anal 1993;13:25–36.

17. Filser JW, Bolt HM. Pharmacokinetics of halogenated ethylenes in rats. Arch Toxicol 1979;42:123–136.

18. Andersen ME, Gargas ML, Jones RA, Jenkins LJ. Determination of the kinetic constants for metabolism of inhaled toxicants in vivo based on gas uptake measurements. Toxicol Appl Pharmacol 1980;54:100–116.

19. Gargas ML, Andersen ME. Determining kinetic constants of chlorinated ethane metabolism in the rat from rates of exhalation. Toxicol Appl Pharmacol 1989;99:344–353.

20. Gargas ML, Andersen ME, Clewell HJ III. A physiologically based simulation approach for determining metabolic constants from gas uptake data. Toxicol Appl Pharmacol 1986;86:341–352.

21. Krishnan K, Andersen ME. *In vitro* toxicology and risk assessment. Alt Methods Toxicol 1993;9:185–203.

22. Bisgaard HC, Lam HR. In vitro and in vivo studies on the metabolism of 1,3-diaminobenzene: comparison of metabolites formed by the perfused rat liver, primary rat hepatocyte cultures, hepatic rat microsomes and the whole rat. Toxicol In Vitro 1989;3:167–174.

23. Reitz RH, Mendrala AL, Guengereich FP. *In vitro* metabolism for methylene chloride in human and animal tissues: Use in physiologically-based pharmacokinetic models. Toxicol Appl Pharmacol 1989;97:230–246.

24. Reitz RH, Gargas ML, Mendrala AL, Schumann AM. *In vivo* and *in vitro* studies of perchloroethylene metabolism for physiologically based pharmacokinetic modeling in rats, mice, and humans. Toxicol Appl Pharmacol 1996;136:289–306.

25. Kedderis GL, Fennell TR. Development of a physiologically based description of acrylonitrile dosimetry. CIIT Activities 1996;16:1–8.

26. Reitz RH, Gargas ML, Andersen ME, Provan WM, Green TL. Predicting cancer risk from vinyl chloride exposure with a physiologically based pharmacokinetic model. Toxicol Appl Pharmacol 1996;137:253–267.

27. Kotin P, Falk H, Busser R. Distribution, retention and elimination of ^{14}C-3,4-benzpyrene after administration to mice and rats. J Natl Cancer Inst 1959;24:541–555.
28. Schlede E, Kuntzman R, Haber S, Conney AH. Effect of enzyme induction on the metabolism and tissue distribution of benzo(a)pyrene. Cancer Res 1970;30: 2893–2897.
29. Wiersma DA, Roth RA. The prediction of benzo(a)pyrene clearance by rat liver and lung from enzyme kinetic data. Mol Pharmacol 1983;24:300–308.
30. Roth RA, Vinegar A. Action by the lungs on circulating xenobiotic agents, with a case study of physiologically based pharmacokinetic modeling of benzo(a)pyrene disposition. Pharmacol Ther 1990;48:143–155.
31. Withey JR, Shedden J, Law FCP, Abedini S. Distribution of benzo(a)pyrene in pregnant rats following inhalation exposure and a comparison with similar data obtained with pyrene. J Appl Toxicol 1993;13:193–202.
32. Haenni EO, Howard JW, Joe FL. Dimethyl sulfoxide: a superior analytical extracting solvent for polynuclear hydrocarbons and for some highly chlorinated hydrocarbons. J Assoc Off Anal Chem 1963;45:67–70.
33. Harrison LI, Gibaldi M. Physiologically based pharmacokinetic model for Digoxin distribution and elimination in the rat. J Pharm Sci 1977;66:1138–1142.
34. Travis CC, Bowers JC. Protein binding of benzene under ambient exposure conditions. Toxicol Ind Health 1989;5:1017–1024.

II CURRENT TRENDS AND FUTURE DIRECTIONS

9 Resources for Biomedical Research
Opportunities for Alternatives

Elaine Young, PhD

The National Center for Research Resources (NCRR) at the National Institutes of Health (NIH) supports infrastructure for the biomedical research community. This infrastructure includes facilities, such as the General Clinical Research Centers and Synchrotron Centers, as well as Research Animal Facilities, such as the regional Primate Centers. The NCRR also provides for researchers to share large, expensive equipment through shared instrumentation grants. Finally, the NCRR supports the distribution of biomaterials and animal models through Comparative Medicine.

Comparative Medicine has a focus in the exploration, development, and distribution of nonmammalian models for research. This focus provides for development of new models or expansion of the use of established models, which are the foundation of medical advances. Resource facilities are supported that develop and provide models for the research community, and are heavily used by investigators who are funded through other NIH Institutes. Approximately 65% of the 1996 budget of $12 million was used to support investigator-initiated research grants and the remaining 35% supported resources.

Resources include the American Type Culture Collection in Rockville, MD, which is dedicated to the acquisition, preservation, authentication, and distribution of living microorganisms and cell lines. The collection distributes over 150,000 of these cultures and cell lines each year.

The Bloomington Drosophila Stock Center in Bloomington, IN, maintains and distributes *Drosophila melanogaster* mutations as well as information associated with this fly. The center, which is jointly

From: *Toxicity Assessment Alternatives: Methods, Issues, Opportunities*
Edited by: H. Salem and S. A. Katz © Humana Press Inc., Totowa, NJ

funded by the NIH and the National Science Foundation, distributes over 26,000 stocks to researchers annually.

The Caenorhabditis Genetics Center in St. Paul, MN, is a repository and distribution center for mutants of the nematode, *Caenorhabditis elegans*. Over 1600 strains are available, and the center also updates and distributes the *C. elegans* genetic map.

The National Cell Culture Center in Minneapolis, MN provides large quantities of animal cells, monoclonal antibodies (MAbs), and nonhybridoma cell-secreted proteins. The center allows researchers to conduct research not possible with the facilities available in their own laboratories.

The National Disease Research Interchange in Philadelphia, PA arranges for retrieval and distribution of normal and diseased human tissues and organs for biomedical researchers. Over 165 different types of human tissue are procured from autopsies, eye banks, surgical procedures, and organ-retrieval programs.

The National Resource for Aplysia in Miami, FL provides a consistent supply of live, healthy *Aplysia californica* from all life stages. The center raises the animal and its food source, and provides investigators with heterozygosity data and genetic markers for certain traits. This model organism was discovered 20 years ago by Eric Kandel *(1)*, and is especially useful for learning and behavior and developmental neurophysiology studies because it has a small number of large identifiable neurons, which have been linked to its behavior.

The National Resource Center for Cephalopods in Galveston, TX provides a consistent supply of live, healthy squids, and other cells, tissue, and organ systems of cephalopods.

The Yeast Genetic Stock Center in Berkeley, CA collects, maintains, and provides strains of the yeast, *Saccharomyces cerevisiae*. The center maintains over 1000 genetically defined strains and updates, and distributes the genetic map of *S. cerevisiae* to researchers. The map is now complete, and consists of 16 chromosomes, 6000 genes, and 12.5 million bp. This is the first eukaryote to be sequenced, and more than one-third of yeast proteins have been found to have counterparts in humans.

The importance of nonmammalian model systems to biomedical research is underscored by a search of the literature. In the field of genetics, one cannot search long before encountering models, such as *C. elegans*, *Drosophila*, and zebrafish, which contributed to advances in knowledge about programmed cell death and gene regulation. *C. elegans* is an important model system for studies of development, cell biology, and neurobiology. It is 1 mm long, has a short life-span, and is transparent, which has allowed researchers to map the fate of its 3000 or so cells. The lineage from egg to adult is known, and the wiring diagram of its 302 neurons has been worked out. This nematode was also instrumental in the Human Genome Project, not only by developing technologies and strategies, but by locating genes that are homologous to human genes. As Nietzsche predicted when he said "Ye have made your way from worm to man, and much within you is still worm," much of human biology resides in the worm. Thirty-two homologs to human disease genes have been identified in *C. elegans* to date, and others are expected when the sequencing is completed in 1997 or 1998.

Drosophila gained worldwide attention as a model last year when the Nobel Prize in medicine went to three researchers who discovered the genes and proteins that form the first specialized structures (eyes) in the fly. Many of these genes have counterparts in humans. Because of the recognition that developmental genes are similar from flies to humans, several biotech firms have been founded to develop drugs that rejuvenate damaged tissues by reactivating the embryonic gene in the adult.

Fish constitute 43% of all vertebrate species, whereas only 12% of vertebrates are mammals. Fish represent the largest group of cold-blooded experimental vertebrates and are rapidly making inroads into the biomedical research laboratory. In particular, the zebrafish, a small, striped fish common to home aquaria, has become the fish of choice for biomedical research on embryological studies. Comparative Medicine is supporting construction of a genetic linkage map, developing a transgenic line, and developing methods to cryopreserve genetic lines of this valuable model. In addition to the advantages offered by the zebrafish of high reproductive rate and the ease of developing mutants, the economics of using the zebrafish as a model are considerable: one finds that one can support 1680 zebrafish for the same cost as 17 mice or one dog.

The value of these and other "nontraditional" model organisms is being recognized by the research community. As a result, it is now possible to gather information on the Internet about availability, care and feeding, current methodologies, and research news of several of these models. NetVet Veterinary Resources (http://netvet.wustl.edu/welctext.ht) provides valuable information on various animal models, including invertebrates, fish, and reptiles. The Fish Net (http://zfish.uoregon.edu/index.html) provides comprehensive information about zebrafish, including an address book of zebrafish researchers. The NCRR homepage (http://www.ncrr.nih.gov) also can be contacted to obtain information about these and other resources funded by NCRR.

REFERENCE

1. Kandel ER, et al. Classical conditioning and sensitization share aspects of the same molecular cascade in Aplysia. Cold Spring Harbor Symp. Quant. Biol. 1983;48:821–830.

III MECHANISTICALLY BASED TEST METHODS AS ALTERNATIVES

10 Endocrine Disruption in Wildlife
Scientific Processes and Principles for Evaluating Effects

Richard Dickerson, PhD, DABT and Ronald Kendall, Sr., PhD

CONTENTS

INTRODUCTION
FORMAT OF MEETING
CONCLUSIONS AND RESEARCH NEEDS
ACKNOWLEDGMENTS
REFERENCES

INTRODUCTION

The discovery that reproductive abnormalities are present in animals born in ecosystems polluted with chemicals known or suspected to have endocrine-disrupting effects may be considered a warning message from wildlife *(1,2)*. Embryonic death, deformities, and abnormal nesting behavior have been observed in fish-eating birds residing in portions of the Great Lakes area where contamination with persistent chlorinated hydrocarbons was known to have occurred *(3,4)*. These hydrocarbons included insecticides, such as 1,1,1-trichloro-2,2-(4-chlorophenyl)-ethane (DDT) and methoxychlor, as well as the polychlorinated and polybrominated biphenyls (PCBs and PBBs). Researchers have observed bald eagles *(Haliaeetus leucocephalus)* with crossed beaks, other cranio-facial abnormalities, and brain asymmetry *(3–5)*. Fish in the Great Lakes have reproductive and thyroid abnormalities, whereas male trout *(Oncorhyncus mykiss)* in some rivers in the UK have elevated plasma vitellogenin levels *(6–9)*. In the Everglades region of Florida,

From: *Toxicity Assessment Alternatives: Methods, Issues, Opportunities*
Edited by: H. Salem and S. A. Katz © Humana Press Inc., Totowa, NJ

panthers *(Felis concolor coryi)* have cryptorchidism and other reproductive abnormalities *(10)*. Also in Florida, American alligators *(Alligator mississippiens)* in Lake Apopka exhibited decreased numbers of juveniles, decreased clutch viability, and abnormalities in reproductive organs following a Dicofol (methoxychlor) spill *(11–13)*. Effects were observed in mink *(Mustela vison)* fed fish from the Great Lakes and in Beluga whales *(Delphinapterus leucas)* of the St. Lawrence River *(14–17)*.

Based on scientific observation, we know that both man-made (DDT/DDE, PCBs/PBBs) and natural compounds (phytoestrogens) have the ability to cause alterations of the endocrine system in both humans and wildlife. We know that these alterations may be reversible or irreversible, and that the effects may be adverse or nonadverse on individuals or populations. In areas that received significant contamination, there is irrefutable evidence of adverse effects on wildlife.

The overriding concern, however, is whether background levels of these same and similar compounds pose a risk to wildlife and human populations. In other words, do these background levels of xenobiotics found in most ecosystems have the potential for causing adverse effects on the endocrine systems of wildlife populations? At the present time, we do not have the database or the methodology for making an informed decision. As a result, we have recently concluded a scientific panel discussion held at Kiawah Island, South Carolina, to develop the processes and principles for conducting a risk-based ecological risk assessment on endocrine disrupting chemicals. This meeting built on scientific principles established in earlier meetings on both wildlife toxicology and endocrine disruption. The panel incorporated researchers from academia, government, and industry. The following information resulted from discussions and conclusions drawn from this meeting.

FORMAT OF MEETING

The meeting began with plenary sessions discussing wildlife conservation, the framework for ecological risk assessment in wildlife (R. Kendall), mechanisms of endocrine disruption (A. Brouwer), and principles for assessing effects on the endocrine system both in the laboratory and in the field (J. Giesy). These were followed by a series of presentations on the principles and processes of ecological risk assessment of endocrine-disrupting chemicals. Presentations included hazard identification/epidemiology (J. Lamb, P. Matthiessen), exposure assessment (D. Tillitt, K. Solomon), mechanisms (T. Zacharewski, G. van der Kraak), dose–response assessment (R. Dickerson, A. Brouwer), wildlife sentinels (D. M. Fry, M. Hooper), weight of evidence (J. Giesy, G. Ankley), and uncertainties (W. Suk, R. Miller).

Next, case studies of chemically induced endocrine disruption were presented and discussed. The remainder of the meeting was devoted to workshops on the principles of risk assessment of endocrine disrupters. The meeting concluded with presentations by the chairs of the breakout sessions *(see above)*. These presentations are summarized in the next section.

Principles of Endocrine Risk Assessment in Wildlife

The principles section of the meeting consisted of an introductory talk by the chair and/or rapporteur of each section, discussion by the subpanel in a breakout session, and development of conclusions. These conclusions are listed below by session topic.

The hazard identification session, chaired by J. Lamb, determined there is a need for better assessment of chemical fate to determine potential exposure. This group believes that current in vitro methods are not sufficiently accurate or broad-based enough to replace apical testing in animals. They suggested that better in vitro and functional binding assays should be developed and validated for chemicals that fall into classes with known endocrine-disrupting activity. They also suggested that multigenerational testing needs to be performed in avian species and reptiles or amphibians, in addition to the mandated multigenerational testing in mammals. Finally, this group emphasized that many of the tests required for effective testing have not yet been developed and that this is a deterrent to the development of an effective testing strategy.

The exposure session, chaired by D. Tillitt, examined current exposure assessment techniques and concluded that chemical residue analysis methods are satisfactory in terms of technology, but need to be coupled with biomarkers of exposure that are relevant for endocrine disrupters. Biomarkers that are capable of detecting both exposure and effects are particularly useful. It is also necessary to know the rate at which the body burden was accumulated. A slow gradual exposure of a lipophilic chemical allows the compound to be deposited in the fat without eliciting adverse effects on the exposed animal, whereas a higher exposure over a shorter time period may result in similar levels measured in the fat, but may elicit adverse effects in the exposed organism. Moreover, they emphasized the importance of the timing of the exposure. Exposure to adult animals is likely to result in other adverse effects before reproductive or other endocrine effects become evident *(18)*. In contrast, exposure during fetal development, the period immediately after birth, or during puberty can result in severe reproductive or developmental effects in the absence of overt toxicity *(19–21)*.

The mechanisms session, chaired by T. Zacharewski, developed a clear definition of endocrine disrupters, and selected chemicals to use as models for endocrine disrupters that affect hormonal synthesis and catabolism, secretion and transport of hormones, and nuclear membrane mechanisms. This group also examined the limitations and predictive value of in vitro assays. In particular, the use of proliferation assays in human breast cancer cell lines is insufficient in that compounds that cause proliferation are not necessarily acting through the endocrine system. In vitro systems that are mechanistically based are in the process of implementation and will eliminate some of the limitations of earlier in vitro systems. These include mammalian and yeast cell lines that have reporter genes coupled to response elements for the various hormone receptors *(22,23)*. It will be necessary to determine the degree of concordance between these assays and the results observed in vivo.

The dose–response assessment session, chaired by R. Dickerson, defined the difference between endocrine disrupters and endocrine modulators. The difficulty of selecting appropriate end points when multiple target sites exist, compounded by the presence of both endogenous and exogenous ligands, and multiple mechanisms of action occurring simultaneously was the discussion focus of this group. The importance of the shape of the dose–response curve, mixtures, and environmentally relevant concentrations were also the subject of spirited discussion. The overall conclusion reached was that endocrine-disrupting chemicals require a more complex risk-assessment paradigm than do chemicals that have single target sites.

The wildlife sentinels session, chaired by M. Fry, examined the characteristics of good wildlife sentinels, and considered the question of how many sentinels and at what trophic levels are required. This group also explored what the characteristics of good wildlife sentinels may be. The problem of what to do in an ecological risk assessment when the sentinel species possesses exquisite sensitivity to the chemical of concern was also a point of discussion.

The weight of evidence session, chaired by J. Giesy, considered the relevance of in vitro data in predicting in vivo effects, the possibility of latent effects, and the question of which end points in how many species need to be measured for any degree of confidence. The framework for conducting assessments of endocrine-disrupting chemicals was also debated.

The uncertainties session, chaired by W. Suk, considered uncertainties in the following areas: effects elicited by relevant environmental mixtures, in the ability to extrapolate between wildlife species and between wildlife and humans, and into how much endocrine insult may be borne by wildlife without influencing survivability and reproduction.

Case Study Examples

Case studies involving endocrine disruption in wildlife were presented and then discussed by the expert panel. The case studies were divided into four areas: fish, birds, reptiles, and mammals. Certain classes of industrial chemicals have caused vitellogenin production in male fish and cytochrome P450 induction. These effects are pronounced during periods of low stream flow. In the fish study, P. Matthiessen reported to the group on the estrogenic effects on trout living in rivers downstream of effluent outfalls. Feminization of male trout, characterized by the production of vitellogenin in male fish, was observed at several sites. The degree of effect was influenced by the season of the year and the flow rate of the stream receiving the effluent. The exact causal nature of the feminization was not stated; however, possible candidates include nonylphenols and pharmaceutical steroids among others. After Matthiessen's presentation, G. van der Kraak discussed the effects of phytoestrogens on fish. Bleached Kraft paper mill effluent (BKME) contains numerous lignins that become chlorinated during the process of making paper and are released into the effluent. Compounds in this complex mixture may have estrogenic or anti-estrogenic properties, and can cause perturbations of the pituitary–gonadal axis at several locations.

In birds, D. M. Fry's case study dealt with a historical perspective of exposure of avian species to chlorinated hydrocarbons. This was followed by a presentation on the present status of avian species residing in the Great Lakes by Gary Heinz. It is clear that exposure to DDT and its metabolites as well as the PCBs had toxic effects on raptors and piscivorous birds in the late 1960s and early 1970s. Effects, such as egg shell thinning, sexual role reversal, embryo death, and abnormalities, including cranio-facial deformations, led to major effects on populations in certain areas where exposure was high. Since the banning of DDT and PCBs, many bird populations have rebounded in most areas of the Great Lakes. Widespread use of DDT resulted in reduction of bald eagle populations in the Great Lakes owing to egg shell thinning. Once the use of DDT was banned, and environmental levels began to fall, it became apparent that PCBs were adversely affecting eagle health as well (24–26). Effects included developmental abnormalities, such as cranio-facial deformities and reproductive effects. The use of PCBs was banned in the 1970s, and environmental levels of this class of compounds is steadily decreasing as well. The incidence of developmental and reproductive abnormalities in eagles and other fish-eating birds appears to be declining and the populations of the affected species are rebounding.

J. Bergeron discussed the effects of hydroxylated PCBs on turtles, whereas W. Rhodes gave a presentation on the health of the alligator populations in the state of South Carolina. It is known that certain PCBs can be hydroxylated to produce products that are estrogenic *(27)*. Administration of these hydroxylated PCB to turtle eggs results in the internalization of the hydroxylated PCBs and binding to the estrogen receptor of the developing embryo. If this occurs during the period of organogenesis of the gonad, eggs incubated at male-producing tempera-tures produce female hatchlings. However, the PCBs that are estrogenic when hydroxylated at the 4' position are only a minor constituent of the PCBs found in the environment. The effects elicited by the hydroxy-lated PCBs, when present in high enough concentrations, are similar to those observed by Guillette and coworkers at Lake Apopka in Florida *(12,13,28,29)*. These finding cause concern for the populations of rep-tiles utilizing temperature-dependent sex determination. It does not appear, however, that background levels of these and other endocrine active chemicals are high enough to affect alligator populations in gen-eral. Walt Rhodes, of South Carolina Department of Natural Resources, believes that throughout most of their range, alligator populations are habitat-limited. Young females are driven off nesting sites by the older females resulting in egg absorption. The populations have reached the nuisance level in several southern states, resulting in the establishment of hunting seasons in Florida, Louisiana, South Carolina, and Texas.

The last case study dealt with endocrine disruption in mammals and was discussed by J. Giesy and J. Stegeman. John Giesy discussed research into the effects of PCBs on mink reproduction. If concentra-tions of PCBs are high enough in fish used as a food supply, reproduc-tive failure occurs in the mink with early fetal death as noted by postpartum placental sites *(14,15,30)*. In addition, the kits exposed to fish from the Great Lakes had decreased survival and lower body weights as compared to controls. Analysis of the Great Lakes fish (carp) used as a food supply shows that levels of mercury, total PCBs, 2,3,7,8-tetra-chlorodibenzo-*p*-dioxin equivalents (TCDD-EQ), DDT, as well as other organochlorine pesticides were elevated as compared to fish from waters above the dams leading into the Great Lakes *(3)*.

Studies in free-ranging dolphins have demonstrated that decreased lymphocyte responses are correlated with elevated concentrations of both organochlorine insecticides (predominantly DDT) and PCB con-centrations in venous blood *(31)*. This decrease in immune function may be related to recently observed incidences of strandings and unusual mortality. Beluga whales inhabiting the St. Lawrence seaway also have elevated body burdens of contaminants and show increased incidence of tumors *(17,32)*. Necropsy of stranded whales showed functional and morphological changes in the thyroid and the adrenal cortex. Moreover, the population appears to be dwindling. Numbers of whales around the turn of the century approached 5000, whereas current estimates are between 400 and 500 whales. A possible explanation is organochlorine-contaminated-induced immune suppression resulting in a failure of tumor surveillance and increased incidence of mortality from bacterial and/or viral infection. Uterine occlusions and decreased reproductive success have been observed in harbor seals *(Phoca vitulina)* of the Dutch Wadden Sea; these effects were correlated with increasing PCB levels in the adipose tissue *(33)*.

CONCLUSIONS AND RESEARCH NEEDS

The following conclusions evolved from discussions and panel recommendations: (1) It is clear, from the case studies in wildlife evaluated at this meeting and the mechanistic discussions that followed, that certain environmental chemicals, including parent compounds and metabolites, have the potential to disrupt the endocrine system in wildlife. This conclusion is substantiated by current scientific information. (2) It is obvious that in areas that received extensive chemical contamination, such as the Great Lakes region of North America, Lake Apopka, and regions of coastal southern California, when exposure is high, disruptions in the reproduction and/or health of wildlife have occurred. However, the more generalized effects in a broad range of wildlife and their populations at a national or global scale are not clearly apparent at this time and will require more research to evaluate "cause and effect," and potential impacts on survival and reproduction. The scientific database on endocrine effects in wildlife is nowhere near complete and continues to evolve. Continuing efforts to utilize a risk-based approach that incorporates a better understanding of exposure as well as effects at both the individual and population levels are warranted *(34,35)*.

We are moving forward in this area aggressively. We have completed or in the process of completing three means of disseminating the compilation of information from this conference:

1. "A letter to the editors" of the journal *Environmental Toxicology and Chemistry*, describing the purpose and the agenda of the Kiawah meeting. This was published in volume 15, issue 8, pages 1253–1254.
2. A special symposium dealing with endocrine effects in wildlife at the annual meeting of the Society of Environmental Toxicology and Chemistry was held in Washington, DC in November of 1996. The symposium lasted for two days and covered basic science, field studies, and

risk assessment. The symposium was chaired by G. Ankley, R. Dickerson, S. Smith, and R. Kendall. The proceedings of the Symposium were published as Vol. 17, No. 1, of *Environmental Toxicology and Chemistry*, January 1998.

3. A book entitled *Processes and Principles for Evaluating Endocrine Disruption in Wildlife*, edited by R. J. Kendall, R. L. Dickerson, J. P. Giesy, and W. Suk. This book was released in March of 1998.

ACKNOWLEDGMENTS

The meeting and resulting publications were facilitated by ECORISK, Inc., the Chemical Manufacturer's Association, and NIEHS.

REFERENCES

1. Colborn T. The wildlife/human connection: modernizing risk decisions. Environ Health Perspectives 1994;102:55–59.
2. Leblanc GA. Are environmental sentinels signaling? Environ Health Perspectives 1995;103:888–890.
3. Giesy JP, Ludwig JP, Tillitt DE. Dioxins, dibenzofurans, PCBs and colonial fish-eating water birds. In: Schecter A, ed., Dioxins and Health. Plenum, New York, 1994, pp. 254–307.
4. Fry DM. Reproductive effects in birds exposed to pesticides and industrial chemicals. Environ Health Perspectives 1995;103:165–171.
5. Henshel DS, Martin JW, Norstrom R, Whitehead P, Steeves JD, Cheng KM. Morphometric abnormalities in brains of great blue heron hatchlings exposed in the wild to PCDDs. Environ Health Perspectives 1995;103:61–66.
6. Sumpter JP. Feminized responses in fish to environmental estrogens. Toxicol Lett 1995;82:737–742.
7. Purdom CE, Hardiman PA, Bye VJ, Eno NC, Tyler CR, Sumpter JP. Estrogenic effects of effluents from sewage treatments works. Chem Ecol 1994; 8:275–285.
8. MacLatchy DL, Van Der Kraak GJ. The phytoestrogen beta-sitosterol alters the reproductive endocrine status of goldfish. Toxicol Appl Pharmacol 1995;134: 305–312.
9. Bortone SA, Davis WP. Fish intersexuality as indicator of environmental stress. Bioscience 1994;44:165–172.
10. Facemire CF, Gross TS, Guillette LJ. Reproductive impairment in the Florida panther: nature or nurture? Environ Health Perspectives 1995;103:79–86.
11. Crews D, Bergeron JM. Role of reductase and aromatase in sex determination in the red-eared slider *(Trachemys scripta)*, a turtle with temperature-dependent sex determination. J Endocrinol 1994;143:279–289.
12. Guillette LJ, Gross TS, Masson GR, Matter JM, Percival HF, Woodward AR. Developmental abnormalities of the gonad and abnormal sex hormone concentrations in juvenile alligators from contaminated and control lakes in Florida. Environ Health Perspectives 1994;102:680–688.
13. Guillette LJ, Gross TS, Gross DA, Rooney AA, Percival HF. Gonadal steroidogenesis *in vitro* from juvenile alligators obtained from contaminated or control lakes. Environ Health Perspectives 1995;103:31–36.

14. Heaton SN, Bursian SJ, Giesy JP, Tillitt DE, Render JA, Jones PD, et al. Dietary exposure of mink to carp from Saginaw Bay, Michigan. 1. Effects on reproduction and survival, and the potential risks to wild mink populations. Arch Environ Contam Toxicol 1995;28:334–343.

15. Tillitt DE, Gale RW, Meadows JC, Zajicek JL, Peterman PH, Heaton SN, et al. Dietary Exposure of mink to carp from Saginaw Bay. 3. Characterization of dietary exposure to planar halogenated hydrocarbons, dioxin equivalents, and bio-magnification. Environ Sci Technol 1996;30:283–291.

16. DeGuise S, Lagace A, Beland P. Tumors in St. Lawrence beluga whales *(Delphinapterus leucas)*. Vet Pathol 1994;31:444–449.

17. DeGuise S, Martineau D, Beland P, Fournier M. Possible mechanisms of action of environmental contaminants on St. Lawrence beluga whales *(Delphinapterus leucas)*. Environ Health Perspectives 1995;103:73–77.

18. Johnson L, Safe S, Dickerson R. Effect of 2,3,7,8-tetrachlorodibenzo-p-dioxin on spermatogenesis and Leydig cell volume in adult rats. Chemosphere 1992; 25:1175–1181.

19. Mably TA, Moore RW, Peterson RE. *In utero* and lactational exposure of male rats to 2,3,7,8-tetrachlordibenzo-p-dioxin. 1: Effects on androgenic status. Toxicol Appl Pharmacol 1992;114:97–107.

20. Mably TA, Moore RW, Goy RW, Peterson RE. *In utero* and lactational exposure of male rats to 2,3,7,8-tetrachlordibenzo-p-dioxin. 2: Effects on sexual behavior and the regulation of luteinizing hormone secretion in adulthood. Toxicol Appl Pharmacol 1992;114:108–117.

21. Mably TA, Bierke DL, Moore RW, Gendron-Fitzpatrick A, Peterson RE. *In utero* and lactational exposure of male rats to 2,3,7,8-tetrachlordibenzo-p-dioxin. 3: Effects on spermatogenesis and reproductive capability. Toxicol Appl Pharmacol 1992;114:118–126.

22. Balaguer P, Joyeux A, Denison MS, Vincent R, Gillesby BE, Zacharewski T. Assessing the estrogenic and dioxin-like activities of chemicals and complex mixtures using *in vitro* recombinant receptor-reporter gene assays. Can J Physiol Pharmacol 1996;74:216–222.

23. Murk AJ, Boudewijn TJ, Meininger PL, Bosveld ATC, Rossaert G, Ysebaert T, et al. Effects of polyhalogenated aromatic hydrocarbons and related contaminants on common tern reproduction: integration of biological, biochemical and chemical data. Arch Environ Contam Toxicol 1996;31:128–140.

24. Boden SD, Joyce ME, Oliver B, Heydemann A, Bolander ME. Estrogen receptor messenger RNA expression in callus during fracture healing in the rat. Calcif Tissue Int 1989;45:324–325.

25. Bowerman, WW IV, Best DA, Kubiak TJ, Giesy JP, Sikarskie JG. The influence of environmental contaminants on bald eagle *(Haliaeetus leucocephalus)* populations in the Laurentian Great Lakes, North America. In: Meyburg BU, Chancellor RD, eds. Raptor Conservation Today. Pica Press, East Sussex, Great Britain, 1994, pp. 703–707.

26. Bowerman WW, Giesy JP, Best DA, Kramer VJ. A review of factors affecting productivity of bald eagles in the Great Lakes region: implications for recovery. Environ Health Perspectives 1995;103:51–59.

27. Korach KS, Sarver P, Chae K, McLachlan JA, McKinney JD. Estrogen receptor-binding activity of polychlorinated hydroxybiphenyls: conformationally restricted structural probes. Mol Pharmacol 1988;33:120–126.

28. Guardino X, Serra C, Obiols J, Rosell MG, Berenguer MJ, Lopez F, et al. Determination of DDT and related compounds in blood samples from agricultural workers. J Chromatog 1996;719:141–147.

29. Guillette LJ, Pickford DB, Crain DA, Rooney AA, Percival HF. Reduction in penis size and plasma testosterone concentrations in juvenile alligators living in a contaminated environment. Gen Comp Endocrinol 1996;101:32–42.
30. Backlin BM, Bergman A. Histopathology of postpartum placental sites in mink *(Mustela vison)* exposed to polychlorinated biphenyls or fractions thereof. APMIS 1995;103:843–854.
31. Lahvis GP, Wells RS, Kuehl DW, Stewart JL, Rhinehart HL, Via CS. Decreased lymphocyte responses in free-ranging bottlenose dolphins *(Tursiops truncatus)* are associated with increased concentrations of PCBs and DDT in peripheral blood. Environ Health Perspectives 1995;103:67–72.
32. Beland P, Blakely B, Boermans H, Boileau S, De Guise S, Fournier M, et al. 1994. Markers of organohalogen toxicity in St. Lawrence Beluga whales. Final Report. Toxen Biological Sciences, St. Lawrence National Institute of Ecotoxicology, Montreal, Canada.
33. Oehme M, Furst P, Kruger C, Meemken HA, Groebel W. Presence of polychlorinated dibenzo-p-dioxin, dibenzofurans and pesticides in Artic seal from Spitzbergen. Chemosphere 1988;17:1291–1300.
34. Dickerson RL, Hooper MJ, Gard NW, Cobb GP, Kendall RJ. Toxicological foundations of ecological risk assessment: biomarker development and interpretation based on laboratory and wildlife species. Environ Health Perspectives 1994;102: 65–69.
35. Kendall RJ, Lacher TE, Bunck C, Daniel B, Driver C, Grue CE, et al. An ecological risk assessment of lead shot exposure in non-waterfowl avian species: upland game birds and raptors. Environ Toxicol Chem 1996;15:4–20.

11 Mechanistic Animal-Replacement Approaches for Predicting Pharmacokinetics of Organic Chemicals

Patrick Poulin, PHD, Martin Beliveau, BSc, and Kannan Krishnan, PHD

CONTENTS

INTRODUCTION
MECHANISTIC ANIMAL-REPLACEMENT APPROACHES
    FOR PREDICTING PCS
MECHANISTIC ANIMAL-REPLACEMENT APPROACHES
    FOR PREDICTING BIOCHEMICAL PARAMETERS
REFERENCES

INTRODUCTION

The prediction of the pharmacokinetic behavior of chemicals prior to experimentation in animals and humans is a major challenge. Physiologically based pharmacokinetic (PBPK) models represent a useful framework for simulating the tissue and blood concentration profiles of chemicals in intact animals and humans for various exposure scenarios, routes, and dose levels *(1)*. The PBPK models refer to mathematical descriptions of absorption, distribution, metabolism, and elimination of chemicals in biota based on proven/hypothetical interrelationships among certain mechanistic determinants *(2,3)*. The basic mechanistic determinants included in PBPK models are the physiological characteristics (e.g., cardiac output, alveolar ventilation rate, tissue volumes,

From: *Toxicity Assessment Alternatives: Methods, Issues, Opportunities*
Edited by: H. Salem and S. A. Katz © Humana Press Inc., Totowa, NJ

Table 1
Examples of Physiologically Based Descriptions Used in PBPK Models of VOCs

End points	Equations[a]
Arterial blood concentration	$C_a = [Q_p * C_i + Q_c * C_v]/[Q_p + (Q_c/P_{b:a})]$
Venous blood concentration	$C_v = [\sum_{t=1}^{n} Q_t C_{vt})]/Q_c$
Tissue concentration	
Nonmetabolizing tissues	$C_t = [\int_0^t Q_t * (C_a - C_{vt})]/V_t$
Metabolizing tissues	$C_t = \int_0^t [Q_t * (C_a - C_{vt}) - [V_{max} * C_{vt}/(K_m + C_t)]]/V_t$

[a]C, Q, $P_{b:a}$, V, V_{max}, and K_m refer to concentration, flow rate, blood:air partition coefficient, volume, maximum velocity of metabolism, and metabolism affinity constant. Subscripts a, p, i, c, v, vt, and t refer to arterial blood, alveolar ventilation, inhaled air, cardiac blood flow, mixed venous blood, venous blood leaving tissue, and tissue, respectively.

tissue blood flow rates), biochemical parameters (e.g., maximal velocity and affinity for metabolism), and physicochemical parameters (e.g., blood:air partition coefficients [PCs], tissue:blood PCs, dermal permeability coefficients), which together determine the pharmacokinetic behavior of chemicals in biota (Table 1).

For constructing PBPK models, numerical values of the physiological, physicochemical, and biochemical parameters need to be known. The values of physiological parameters for several species are available in the biomedical literature (1). However, the physicochemical and biochemical parameters need to be determined in vivo or in vitro for each chemical (1,4–6). Alternatively, these parameters can be predicted using animal-replacement approaches. The most commonly used approach in this regard involves the development of empirical equations relating the values of these parameters (e.g., PCs [7–35], dermal permeability coefficient [4,36–53], and biochemical rate constants [8,54–64]) to some other basic chemical-specific parameter, such as the log n-octanol: water partition coefficient or molecular connectivity indices. Following the incorporation of this kind of equation within PBPK models, the numerical values of PCs and biochemical parameters for members of homologous series of chemicals have been obtained and, in turn, used to simulate their pharmacokinetics in animals [65,66]. This approach is essentially a "fitting" exercise that requires collection of extensive experimental data, and its usefulness is limited to the class of compounds for which the data are initially collected. It would be more useful to develop animal-replacement approaches that can provide the numerical values of PBPK model parameters regardless of chemical class. Such approaches should essentially be based on an understanding of the mechanistic determinants of the input parameters required for PBPK modeling.

This chapter presents mechanistic animal-replacement approaches for predicting certain chemical-specific input parameters of PBPK models, namely PCs and biochemical parameters, and their application to predict in vivo pharmacokinetics of organic chemicals.

MECHANISTIC ANIMAL-REPLACEMENT APPROACHES FOR PREDICTING PCS

The PCs refer to the ratio of chemical concentration in two phases (e.g., tissue and air, blood and air, tissue and blood) at equilibrium. In general terms, the partitioning of a chemical between two matrices can be predicted if its solubility and binding in each of the two matrices can be estimated with reasonable accuracy. Using this basic premise, mechanistic animal-replacement approaches for predicting tissue:air, blood:air, and tissue:blood PCs have been developed.

Tissue:Air PCs

Tissue:air PCs of low-mol-wt volatile organic chemicals (VOCs), for which macromolecular binding is negligible, can be calculated based on the following general equation *(12,67,68)*:

$$P_{t:a} = (P_{l:a} * V_{lt}) + (P_{w:a} * V_{wt}) \tag{1}$$

where $P_{l:a}$ = lipid:air partition coefficient, $P_{w:a}$ = water:air partition coefficient, V = volume of tissue components, namely, lipids (lt) and water (wt).

In the above equation, $P_{l:a}*V_{lt}$ represents the partitioning of a chemical between tissue lipids and air, and $P_{w:a}*V_{wt}$ represents the partitioning between tissue water and air. In this context, $P_{o:a}$ (oil:air or n-octanol:air PCs) of chemicals have been used as a surrogate for $P_{l:a}$, and $P_{w:a}$, the reciprocal of Henry's law constant, has been used as a surrogate of chemical partitioning between tissue water and air *(12,67,68)*. Tissue lipids, in fact, represent both neutral (e.g., triglycerides) and polar lipids (e.g., phospholipids). Therefore, the partitioning of a chemical into neutral and polar lipids needs to be considered separately. The physicochemical properties of phospholipids are dependent

Table 2
Average Water and Lipid Levels in Rat Tissues[a]

Tissues	Water	Phospholipids	Neutral lipids
Liver	0.70	0.025	0.035
Muscle	0.74	0.010	0.009
Adipose	0.12	0.002	0.853

[a]Data, expressed as fraction of tissue weight, were obtained from Poulin and Krishnan (70).

on the presence of hydrophobic (e.g., glyceride) and hydrophilic (e.g., phosphomonoester) groups. Therefore, using n-octanol or water-solubility information alone to predict chemical solubility in tissue phospholipids may not be appropriate. Poulin and Krishnan (69,70) proposed the following equation to predict $P_{t:a}$ of VOCs, considering separately the partitioning into neutral and polar lipids:

$$P_{t:a} = (P_{o:a}V_{nt}) + (0.3P_{o:a}V_{pt}) + (0.7P_{w:a}V_{pt}) + (P_{w:a}V_{wt}) \qquad (2)$$

where V_{nt} = volume fraction of neutral lipids, and V_{pt} = volume fraction of phospholipids in tissue, t.

In the above equation, the partitioning of a chemical between tissue neutral lipids and air corresponds directly to $P_{o:a}$, whereas the partitioning between tissue water and air is set equal to $P_{w:a}$. However, the partitioning of a chemical between polar lipids (i.e., phospholipids) and air is calculated as a fractional additive function of the partitioning into neutral lipids ($0.3*P_{o:a}$) and water ($0.7*P_{w:a}$). The latter method of approximation of chemical partitioning into tissue phospholipids is based on the assumption that the lipophilicity-hydrophilicity characteristic of tissue phospholipids is similar to that of commercial lecithin (71,72). According to Eq. 2, $P_{t:a}$ can be calculated with knowledge of tissue composition data, $P_{o:a}$ and $P_{w:a}$. Species-specific data on tissue composition are available in the literature (Table 2). The $P_{o:a}$ and $P_{w:a}$ values for a number of chemicals can be obtained from the literature (7,10,12,16,73). However, it is easier to obtain n-octanol:water or oil:water ($P_{o:w}$) values than $P_{o:a}$ values from the literature. To use the $P_{o:w}$ values rather than $P_{o:a}$, which are not available frequently, Eq. 2 can be rewritten as follows (70):

$$P_{t:a} = [P_{o:w}\,P_{w:a}\,(V_{nt} + 0.3V_{pt})] + [P_{w:a}(V_{wt} + 0.7V_{pt})] \qquad (3)$$

Equations 2 and 3 have been used to predict rat and human $P_{t:a}$ (liver, muscle, fat) of several VOCs (69,70,74–76). In general, the $P_{t:a}$ values

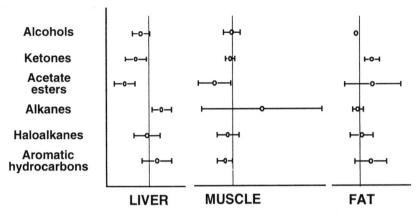

Fig. 1. Ratio of predicted/experimental rat liver:air (l), muscle:air (m), and fat:air (f) PCs for alcohols (l: 0.84 ± 0.22, m: 0.99 ± 0.2, f: 0.91 ± 0.07, $n = 6$), ketones (l: 0.72 ± 0.25, m: 0.96 ± 0.11, f: 1.27 ± 0.17, $n = 5$), acetate esters (l: 0.45 ± 0.25, m: 0.59 ± 0.39, f: 1.29 ± 0.66, $n = 6$), alkanes (l: 1.33 ± 0.2, m: 1.6 ± 1.2, f: 1.02 ± 0.12, $n = 3$), haloalkanes (l: 0.99 ± 0.3, m: 0.9 ± 0.25, f: 1.03 ± 0.27, $n = 17$), and some aromatic hydrocarbons (l: 1.22 ± 0.35, m: 0.81 ± 1.18, f: 1.25 ± 0.38, $n = 7$). Data from Poulin and Krishnan *(69)*. Vertical lines correspond to a ratio of predicted/experimental PCs of 1 for each tissue.

predicted using the animal-replacement approaches were within a factor of two of the experimental data (Fig. 1). $P_{o:w}$ in Eq. 3 refers to *n*-octanol:water PCs or vegetable oil:water PCs of chemicals. In general, *n*-octanol and vegetable oil have been considered useful surrogates of biotic neutral lipids *(12,77,78)*. However, systematic differences between *n*-octanol:water PCs and oil:water PCs are observed for relatively hydrophilic VOCs (i.e., alcohols, acetate esters, ketones), but this is not the case for relatively lipophilic VOCs (i.e., alkanes, haloalkanes, aromatics) *(69,70,77)*. *n*-Octanol, being an alcohol, would appear to solubilize other hydrophilic organics to a greater extent than do biotic neutral lipids. Based on the hydrophilicity-lipophilicity characteristics and the fatty acid composition, vegetable oil has been suggested to be an acceptable alternative to *n*-octanol as a surrogate of biotic neutral lipids, especially for hydrophilic organics *(77)*. Then, to predict $P_{t:a}$ of hydrophilic VOCs, especially for fatty tissues, the $P_{o:w}$ in Eq. 3 should represent vegetable oil:water PCs. However, in the case of relatively lipophilic VOCs (log $P_{o:w}$ > 1.25), there is no difference concerning whether *n*-octanol:water PCs or vegetable oil:water PCs are used as the biotic lipid surrogates *(69,70,77)*.

Tables 3–5 compare the predictions of adipose tissue:air, liver:air, and muscle:air PCs of several other chemicals obtained using the mechanistic

Table 3
Predicted and Experimental Rat Adipose Tissue:Air PCs

Chemicals	Predicted PCs[a]	Experimental PCs[b]
Methanes		
Difluoromethane	4	1.43 ± 0.31
Fluorochloromethane	19	15.4 ± 1
Bromochloromethane	309	325 ± 3
Dibromomethane	819	792 ± 14
Chlorodibromomethane	2291	1917 ± 165
Ethanes		
Chloroethane	33	38.6 ± 0.7
Hexachloroethane	4281	3321 ± 193
1,2-Dibromoethane	1091	1219 ± 50
1-Bromo-2-chloroethane	487	959 ± 39
1,1,1-Trifluoro-2-chloroethane	21	21.2 ± 0.6
1,1,1-Trifluoro-2-bromo-2-chloroethane	169	182 ± 5
Propanes		
1-Chloropropane	90	118 ± 2
2-Chloropropane	60	68.4 ± 2
1,2-Dichloropropane	366	499 ± 30
n-Propyl bromide	232	235 ± 6
Isopropyl bromide	140	158 ± 5
1-Nitropropane	907	506 ± 33
2-Nitropropane	558	155 ± 4
Ethylenes		
Vinyl chloride	21	20 ± 0.7
1,1-Dichloroethylene	55	68.6 ± 2.1
Vinyl bromide	48	49.2 ± 1.3
Aromatics		
Chlorobenzene	1868	1277 ± 43
m-Methyl styrene	12553	11951 ± 692
p-Methyl styrene	11901	11221 ± 972
Others		
Isoflurane	67	98.1 ± 4.6
Allyl chloride	93	101 ± 2
Tricyclodecane	11071	10139 ± 239

[a]Calculated using data on rat tissue composition *(70)*, $P_{o:w}$, and $P_{w:a}$ values *(7)* in Eq. 3.
[b]Experimental data determined under in vitro conditions were obtained from the literature *(7)*.

animal-replacement approach presented above (Eq. 3), with experimental data collected previously using rat tissues. On average, the predicted rat adipose tissue:air PCs varied by a factor of 1.16 (SD = 0.65, $n = 27$)

Table 4
Predicted and Experimental Rat Liver:Air PCs

Chemicals	Predicted PCs[a]	Experimental PCs[b]
Methanes		
Difluoromethane	1	2.75 ± 0.39
Fluorochloromethane	3	3.44 ± 0.27
Bromochloromethane	22	29.2 ± 0.5
Dibromomethane	51	68.1 ± 1.4
Chlorodibromomethane	119	126 ±1 7.1
Ethanes		
Chloroethane	2	3.61 ± 0.32
Hexachloroethane	214	369 ± 17.5
1,2-Dibromoethane	67	119 ± 4
1-Bromo-2-chloroethane	31	42.8 ± 3.3
1,1,1-Trifluoro-2-chloroethane	1	1.84 ± 0.14
1,1,1-Trifluoro-2-bromo-2-chloroethane	9	7.62 ± 1.2
Propanes		
1-Chloropropane	5	5.18 ± 0.38
2-Chloropropane	4	3.15 ± 0.24
1,2-Dichloropropane	20	24.8 ± 2.4
n-Propyl bromide	13	8.17 ± 0.62
Isopropyl bromide	8	4.41 ± 0.34
1-Nitropropane	46	153 ± 17
2-Nitropropane	98	62.4 ± 1.4
Ethylenes		
Vinyl chloride	1	1.6 ± 0.17
1,1-Dichloroethylene	3	4.42 ± 0.30
Vinyl bromide	3	3.33 ± 0.38
Aromatics		
Chlorobenzene	95	86.3 ± 3
m-Methyl styrene	626	327 ± 23
p-Methyl styrene	594	324 ± 17
Others		
Isoflurane	4	4.07 ± 0.2
Allyl chloride	6	38.9 ± 4.5
Tricyclodecane	551	554 ± 17

[a]Calculated using data on rat tissue composition (70), $P_{o:w}$, and $P_{w:a}$ values (7) in Eq. 3.
[b]Experimental data determined under in vitro conditions were obtained from the literature (7).

from the experimental values. The average ratios of the predicted/experimental values were 0.97 (SD = 0.44) and 0.74 (SD = 0.47) for liver:air and muscle:air PCs, respectively. The rat tissue:air PCs have,

Table 5
Predicted and Experimental Rat Muscle:Air PCs

Chemicals	Predicted PCs[a]	Experimental PCs[b]
Methanes		
Difluoromethane	1	1.44 ± 0.25
Fluorochloromethane	3	2.46 ± 0.52
Bromochloromethane	11	11.1 ± 1.8
Dibromomethane	22	40.5 ± 2
Chlorodibromomethane	38	55.6 ± 0.7
Ethanes		
Chloroethane	1	3.22 ± 0.68
Hexachloroethane	61	75 ± 0.9
1,2-Dibromoethane	28	45.6 ± 3.3
1-Bromo-2-chloroethane	13	25.4 ± 3.1
1,1,1-Trifluoro-2-chloroethane	1	1.23 ± 0.14
1,1,1-Trifluoro-2-bromo-2-chloroethane	3	4.46 ± 0.29
Propanes		
1-Chloropropane	2	2.08 ± 0.66
2-Chloropropane	1	2.04 ± 0.48
1,2-Dichloropropane	7	12 ± 1.1
n-Propyl bromide	4	4.21 ± 0.32
Isopropyl bromide	3	4.12 ± 0.35
1-Nitropropane	14	28.9 ± 6.1
2-Nitropropane	81	29.1 ± 3.3
Ethylenes		
Vinyl chloride	1	2.1 ± 0.45
1,1-Dichloroethylene	1	2.05 ± 0.35
Vinyl bromide	1	2.26 ± 0.13
Aromatics		
Chlorobenzene	28	34 ± 3.9
m-Methyl styrene	178	182 ± 10
p-Methyl styrene	169	183 ± 8
Others		
Isoflurane	1	1.6 ± 0.34
Allyl chloride	3	11 ± 0.20
Tricyclodecane	156	674 ± 19

[a]Calculated using data on rat tissue composition (70), $P_{o:w}$, and $P_{w:a}$ values (7) in Eq. 3.
[b]Experimental data determined under in vitro conditions were obtained from the literature (7).

in general, been used for not only developing rat PBPK models, but also human PBPK models, with the assumption that the tissue:air PCs are species-invariant. However, some previous efforts indicated that the liver:air and adipose tissue:air PCs are comparable between species (rat vs human), whereas the muscle:air PCs are somewhat different *(70,76)*. In this context, it might be useful to undertake a systematic comparison of rat and human muscle:air PCs of VOCs. With the availability of mechanism-based algorithms, it becomes easier to evaluate the impact of species differences in tissue composition on the PCs and pharmacokinetics of chemicals.

Blood:Air PCs

The blood:air PC $(P_{b:a})$ is an important input parameter for PBPK modeling of VOCs. This parameter has been calculated in the past using modified forms of Eq. 1 that require data on the lipid, water, and/or protein contents of whole blood *(11,12,68,78–80)*. Some previous studies *(68,78–80)* lumped together the neutral and polar lipid components of blood during the calculations, and only performed limited validation. Other investigators *(11,12)*, using a semiempirical approach to predict $P_{b:a}$, presented a systematic validation of their results. Based on Eq. 3, Poulin and Krishnan *(70,81)* proposed the following mechanistic animal-alternative approach for predicting $P_{b:a}$ of VOCs that do not bind significantly to blood proteins:

$$P_{b:a} = [P_{o:w} \, P_{w:a} \, (V_{nb} + 0.3V_{pb})] + [P_{w:a} \, (V_{wb} + 0.7V_{pb})] \qquad (4)$$

where V = volume fraction of blood components, and *nb*, *pb*, and *wb* refer to neutral lipids, phospholipids, and water, respectively.

Using Eq. 4, $P_{b:a}$ of VOCs can be calculated with the knowledge of blood composition data, $P_{o:w}$ and $P_{w:a}$. The data on lipid and water levels in rat and human blood are available in the literature *(70,81)* and so are the numerical values of $P_{o:w}$ and $P_{w:a}$ at 37°C for several VOCs *(7,10,12,16,17,73,78–80,82)*. The predictions of $P_{b:a}$ obtained using Eq. 4 are adequate for relatively hydrophilic organics (i.e., alcohols, ketones, acetate esters), but it is not the case for relatively lipophilic VOCs (i.e., alkanes, haloalkanes, and aromatic hydrocarbons) *(70,81)* (Fig. 2). For most alkanes, haloalkanes, and aromatic hydrocarbons, the rat $P_{b:a}$ values obtained using Eq. 4 were lower (60–80%) than the experimental data *(70,81)*. The $P_{b:a}$ of a chemical is a composite number that potentially represents two processes occurring in the blood, namely, solubility and binding. Whereas the solubility is likely to be determined by the neutral lipid, phospholipid, and water components of blood, the binding would appear to be associated with plasma proteins and/or hemoglobin. The underpredictions of $P_{b:a}$ of lipophilic VOCs by Eq. 4 can be explained by the lack of consideration of potential binding of

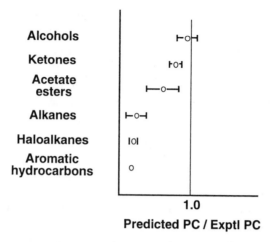

Fig. 2. Ratio of predicted/experimental rat blood:air PCs for alcohols (0.96 ± 0.14), ketones (0.89 ± 0.1), acetate esters (0.63 ± 0.23), alkanes (0.25 ± 0.16), haloalkanes (0.21 ± 0.06), and some aromatic hydrocarbons (0.18 ± 0.03). Data from Poulin and Krishnan *(81)*. The vertical line represents a ratio of predicted/experimental PC of 1.

these chemicals to blood proteins *(81,83,84)*. Larson et al. *(79)* measured under in vitro conditions the hemoglobin:air PCs of halothane, and considered these data during calculations of human $P_{b:a}$. Poulin and Krishnan *(81)* derived the binding association constants (1930 ± 819 M^{-1}) for alkanes, haloalkanes, and aromatic hydrocarbons in rat blood from in vitro experimental data.

Whereas a large discrepancy exists between the experimental values and solubility-based predictions of $P_{b:a}$ (Eq. 4) for relatively lipophilic VOCs, such differences are not apparent in the case of alcohols, ketones, and acetate esters *(81)*. The underestimation of the $P_{b:a}$ of lipophilic VOCs can be explained by possible binding or localization of these chemicals in the hydrophobic pockets of hemoglobin *(81,83,84)*. In order to uncover the determinants of such a process, the lipophilicity characteristics and molecular volumes of several chemicals that have been hypothesized to and not to bind to rat hemoglobin (Table 6) were examined. Figure 3 shows a scatterplot of log $P_{o:w}$ values against geometric volumes of chemicals. The chemicals segregate into two distinct groups, the more leftward group comprising of oxygen-containing chemicals (i.e., ketones, alcohols, acetate esters), and the more rightward group comprising of the oxygen-lacking lipophilic chemicals. Note that VOCs hypothesized to bind to rat hemoglobin are all located within the range limited by a log $P_{o:w}$ value > 1, and a molecular volume < 300 Å^3.

Table 6
Geometric Dimensions (in Angstroms), Oil:Water PCs ($Log\ P_{o:w}$) and Hemoglobin Binding Characteristics of Several Organic Chemicals

Chemicals	$Log\ P_{o:w}$	Length	Width	Depth	Binding[a]
Methyl alcohol	–1.60	5.05	4.73	4.21	–
Ethyl alcohol	–1.29	6.10	4.63	4.21	–
Isopropyl alcohol	–0.99	6.04	5.37	4.75	–
n-Propyl alcohol	–0.79	6.70	5.80	4.12	–
Dimethyl ketone	–0.50	6.10	5.74	4.12	–
n-Butyl alcohol	–0.24	7.98	6.51	4.12	–
Methyl acetate ester	–0.10	7.28	5.64	4.14	–
Methyl ethyl ketone	0.08	7.20	5.74	4.13	–
n-Pentyl alcohol	0.11	9.05	7.46	4.13	–
Ethyl acetate ester	0.39	8.37	6.69	4.13	–
Methyl propyl ketone	0.65	8.49	6.70	4.13	–
Diethyl ether	0.69	7.92	6.69	4.13	–
Isopropyl acetate ester	0.95	8.36	6.73	5.39	–
n-Propyl acetate ester	0.98	9.33	6.77	4.13	–
Methyl chloride	0.99	5.24	4.76	4.58	+
Methyl isobutyl ketone	1.11	7.29	6.21	5.39	–
Dichloromethane	1.34	5.90	5.21	4.12	+
1,2-Dichloroethane	1.51	6.79	6.18	4.12	+
Bromochloromethane	1.62	6.15	5.29	4.12	+
Methyl pentyl ketone	1.62	10.31	8.15	4.13	–
n-Butyl acetate ester	1.69	10.63	7.72	4.13	–
1,1-Dichloroethane	1.88	6.04	5.61	5.27	+
Cis-1,2-dichloroethylene	1.93	6.53	5.33	3.46	+
Chloroform	2.08	6.04	5.61	5.27	+
Trans-1,2-dichloroethylene	2.10	6.51	6.44	3.46	+
Isopentyl acetate ester	2.12	10.63	7.71	5.39	–
1,1,2-Trichloroethane	2.13	6.83	6.22	5.27	+
1,2-Dichloropropane	2.19	7.26	5.75	5.23	+
Benzene	2.23	6.97	6.30	3.54	+
1,1,2,2-Tetrachloroethane	2.43	6.43	6.27	6.04	+
1,1,1-Trichloroethane	2.59	6.43	6.04	5.61	+
Toluene	2.78	7.68	6.97	4.13	+
Trichloroethylene	2.82	6.58	6.52	3.54	+
1,1,1,2-Tetrachloroethane	2.88	6.83	6.43	6.22	+
Chlorobenzene	2.89	7.61	6.97	3.54	+
Carbon tetrachloride	3.03	6.43	6.04	5.90	+
o-Xylene	3.13	7.42	7.39	4.13	+
m-Xylene	3.23	8.31	7.41	4.13	+
p-Xylene	3.27	8.79	7.18	4.13	+
n-Heptane	3.35	11.30	6.11	4.12	+
Styrene	3.40	8.00	7.78	3.54	+
Tetrachloroethylene	3.43	6.63	6.52	3.55	+
Pentachloroethane	3.46	6.87	6.43	6.27	+
n-Hexane	3.78	9.14	7.75	4.13	+
Cyclohexane	4.49	7.00	6.86	5.80	+
Hexachlorobenzene	5.73	9.76	8.93	3.55	–

[a]+, indicates that the hypothesized hemoglobin binding in rats is present. –, signifies the absence of hemoglobin binding for that chemical.

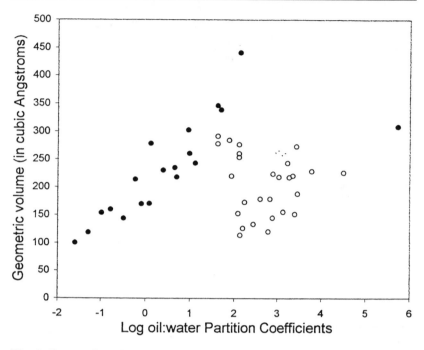

Fig. 3. Geometric volumes and log oil:water PCs of chemicals that have been hypothesized to bind to rat hemoglobin (open circles) and that are not likely to bind to rat hemoglobin (closed circles). Data from Table 6.

Three outliers can be identified in this scheme (methyl isobutyl ketone, n-propyl acetate ester, and isopropyl acetate ester), all of which possess a significant hydrophilic surface (18, 38, and 29%, respectively). The presence of hydrophilic surface is owing to the oxygen atoms contained in these molecules, which may pave the way for hydrogen bond formation, thereby impeding the localization of these substances within the hydrophobic hole in hemoglobin.

It would appear that molecules with

1. Volume >300 Å^3;
2. A log $P_{o:w}$ value < 1; or
3. An oxygen atom in their structure do not bind significantly to hemoglobin, such that solubility-based predictions of $P_{b:a}$ are adequate.

This is supported by the fact that for several alcohols, acetate esters, and ketones, rat $P_{b:a}$ can be adequately predicted only by considering the solubility in blood lipids and water *(81)*. For lipophilic VOCs, however, the binding in blood should be additionally considered *(70)*. For relatively hydrophilic VOCs, human $P_{b:a}$ can be adequately predicted using

Table 7
Average Water and Lipid Levels in Human Blood[a]

Matrices	Water	Phospholipids	Neutral lipids
Whole blood	0.82	0.0024	0.0033
Plasma	0.94	0.0020	0.0032
Erythrocytes	0.63	0.0020	0.0042

[a]Data, expressed as fraction of blood weight, were obtained from Long (85), Nelson (86), and Lentner (87).

blood composition data (Table 7), and $P_{o:w}$ and $P_{w:a}$ values in Eq. 4, i.e., without the consideration of hemoglobin binding (Table 8). Additional data presented in Table 9 confirm that for some of these chemicals, the solubility-based algorithm certainly does not underestimate the components of $P_{b:a}$ (i.e., erythrocyte:air and plasma:air PCs). Since the predicted PC values are only greater and not less than the experimental values, hemoglobin binding of hydrophilic VOCs in humans is not likely to be important, as in the rat (81).

In cases where hemoglobin binding is important, the apparent $P_{b:a}$ can be calculated as follows:

$$P_{b:a(app)} = [C_{a(total)}/C_{air}] \tag{5}$$

where C_a = arterial blood concentration and C_{air} = atmospheric concentration.
Considering the components of $C_{a(total)}$, Eq. 5 can be rewritten as follows:

$$P_{b:a(app)} = [C_{a, free}/C_{air}] + [C_{a, bound}/C_{air}] \tag{6}$$

Since $C_{a, bound} = C_{a, free}K_a C_p/(1 + K_a C_{a, free})$:

$$P_{b:a(app)} = (C_{a, free}/C_{air}) + \{[C_{a, free} * K_a * C_p/C_{air} * (1 + K_a * C_{a, free})]\} \tag{7}$$

where K_a = binding association constant and C_p = concentration of binding proteins. Equation 7 can be rewritten as:

$$P_{b:a(app)} = (C_{a, free}/C_{air}) * [1 + (K_a * C_p)/(1 + K_a * C_{a, free})] \tag{8}$$

The first term of Eq. 8 corresponds to solubility-based $P_{b:a}$ predicted using Eq.4. Therefore, by replacing $C_{a, free}/C_{air}$ with $P_{b:a}$, Eq. 8 reads:

$$P_{b:a(app)} = P_{b:a(pred)} * [1 + (K_a * C_p)/(1 + K_a * C_{a, free})] \tag{9}$$

This equation can be incorporated within PBPK models to calculate the $P_{b,app}$ as a function of time and exposure concentration. Here, the only

Table 8
Predicted and Experimental Human Blood:Air PCs

Chemicals	Predicted PCs[a]	Experimental PCs[b]
Alcohols		
Methanol	2737	1625 – 2590
Ethanol	1759	1265 – 1440
n-Propanol	1521	947 – 1120
Isopropanol	1233	700 – 848
Butanol	1079	677 ± 79
Isobutanol	930	453 – 628
Pentanol	893	534 ± 23
Isopentanol	702	381 ± 16
1-Methoxypropanol	10093	12383 ± 299
1-Methoxyethanol	29475	32836 ± 1350
2-Ethoxyethanol	18959	22093 ± 538
2-Isopropoxyethanol	10153	14416 ± 565
2-Butoxyethanol	5816	7965 ± 61
t-Butyl alcohol	496	462
Acetate esters		
Methyl acetate ester	89	90.1 ± 307
Ethyl acetate ester	59	76.8 ± 3.4
n-Propyl acetate ester	46	73.5 ± 1.7
Isopropyl acetate ester	29	33.1 ± 1.8
Butyl acetate ester	33	83.4 ± 2.9
Isobutyl acetate ester	26	45.1 ± 2.5
n-Pentyl acetate ester	36	92.4 ± 8.4
Isopentyl acetate ester	30	59.1 ± 3
Ethers		
Methyl tertiary ether	13	17.7
Methyl tertiary amyl ether	8	11.7
Ethyl t-butyl ether	11	17.9
Ketones		
Acetone	180	186 ± 20
2-Butanone	96	125 ± 9
Alcenes		
α-Pinene	12	15 ± 4
β-Pinene	17	23 ± 6
3-Carene	20	32 ± 7
Limonene	24	42 ± 8
Aromatics		
1,3-Trimethylbenzene	41	40.8 – 45.2
1,2,4-Trimethylbenzene	42	56.9 – 61.3
1,2,3-Trimethylbenzene	46	63.7 – 69.3

[a]Calculated using average data on human blood composition (84–86), $P_{o:w}$, and $P_{w:a}$ values (10,68,69,80,82,88) in Eq. 4.

[b]Experimental data determined under in vitro conditions were obtained from the literature (9,10,68,80,82,88).

Table 9
Predicted and Experimental Human Erythrocyte:Air and Plasma:Air PCs

Chemicals	Erythrocyte:air PCs		Plasma:air PCs	
	Predicted[a]	Experimental[b]	Predicted[a]	Experimental[b]
Methanol	2106	1522 ± 265	3135	1871 ± 172
Ethanol	1353	1246 ± 215	2015	1455 ± 115
n-Propanol	1171	799 ± 99	1743	969 ± 60
Isopropanol	950	605 ± 68	1413	812 ± 56
Isobutanol	716	519 ± 106	1066	591 ± 154
Acetone	139	170 ± 29	206	217 ± 14
2-Butanone	74	106 ± 10	110	133 ± 11

[a]Calculated using average data on erythrocyte and plasma composition (85–87), $P_{o:w}$, and $P_{w:a}$ values (10,69) in Eq. 4.

[b]Experimental data determined under in vitro conditions were obtained from the literature (9).

additional, chemical-specific parameter that is required relates to K_a. At the present time, there does not exist a validated animal-replacement algorithm for predicting association constants for blood protein binding of organic chemicals. However, based on the analysis presented by Poulin and Krishnan (81), it would appear that the average K_a value for rat hemoglobin binding is 1930 M^{-1} for several VOCs (i.e., chemicals with a molecular volume of <300 Å^3, log $P_{o:w} > 1$, and lacking oxygen in the molecule). This information may be used, at the present time, to provide a first-cut estimate of K_a and $P_{b:a(app)}$ for purposes of PBPK modeling of VOCs in the absence of experimental data.

Tissue:Blood PCs

Tissue:blood PCs ($P_{t:b}$) of VOCs are calculated by dividing the tissue:air PCs with the blood:air PC. For organic chemicals, for which macromolecular binding in tissues and blood is negligible, $P_{t:b}$ can be estimated from $P_{o:w}$ using the following general equation (32,89–92):

$$P_{t:b} = [(P_{o:w}V_{lt} + V_{wt})/(P_{o:w}V_{lb} + V_{wb})] \qquad (10)$$

Some authors considered V_{lt} and V_{lb} in Eq. 10 to represent neutral or total lipid content of tissues and blood, and tested the validity of their approach in a limited manner (32,89,92). Also, they assumed that tissues and blood are constituted exclusively of neutral lipids and water (i.e., $V_{lt} + V_{wt} = 1$) during calculations of $P_{t:b}$ with Eq. 10 (32,89–90,92).

This is unrealistic, considering the fact that some tissues contain as much as 15% protein *(84,86)*. Accounting for differential solubility of chemicals in neutral lipids, phospholipids, and water, and the actual fractional volumes of these components in tissues and blood, Poulin and Krishnan *(70,72,77)* proposed the following algorithm for predicting $P_{t:b}$ of VOCs:

$$P_{t:b} = [P_{o:w} (V_{nt} + 0.3V_{pt}) + (V_{wt} + 0.7V_{pt})]/$$
$$[P_{o:w} (V_{nb} + 0.3V_{pb}) + (V_{wb} + 0.7V_{pb})] \tag{11}$$

The predictions of $P_{t:b}$ obtained using Eq. 11 are identical to the ratio of the predictions of $P_{t:a}$ and $P_{b:a}$ obtained with Eqs. 3 and 4.

The mechanistically based animal-replacement algorithms presented in the preceding paragraphs are useful for predicting PCs of low-mol-wt VOCs required for PBPK modeling. These approaches are also applicable for prediction of $P_{t:b}$s of nonvolatile organic chemicals, which are neither ionized to a significant extent nor bound in the parent chemical form to biological macromolecules *(32)*. In cases where ionization is important, the fraction ionized in the aqueous phase (as a function of the pH of biological fluids) should be taken into account. The consideration of binding to calculate apparent $P_{t:b}$ can be done with knowledge of K_a and C_p. Even though the $P_{t:a}$, $P_{b:a}$, and $P_{t:b}$ of organic chemicals can be predicted using animal-alternative approaches, their pharmacokinetic profiles can be predicted using PBPK framework only if the metabolic rate constants are known.

MECHANISTIC ANIMAL-REPLACEMENT APPROACHES FOR PREDICTING BIOCHEMICAL PARAMETERS

The major constraint for developing PBPK models prior to the conduct of in vitro or in vivo studies in animals and humans relates to reliable prediction of the pathways and rates of biochemical processes in the intact organism. Softwares and expert systems are available for predicting the plausible metabolic pathways and potential metabolites of chemicals *(93–95)*. However, there does not exist a validated methodology for providing quantitative predictions of the chemical-specific metabolic constants (i.e., maximal velocity, V_{max}; Michaelis affinity constant, K_m).

In PBPK models, the rate of hepatic metabolism (RAM) for first-order conditions is often described as follows:

$$RAM = CL_{int} \times C_{vl} \tag{12}$$

where $CL_{int} = V_{max}/K_m$ (L/h) and C_{vl} = chemical concentration in venous blood leaving liver (mg/L).

To solve the above equation, numerical values of V_{max} and K_m, or that of CL_{int} are required. An alternative approach of simulating RAM in PBPK models would involve the use of an equation based on the classical hepatic clearance concept *(96)*, which recognizes the role of blood flow rate in limiting hepatic metabolism. Accordingly, RAM can be calculated with the following alternative forms:

$$\text{RAM} = CL_h \times C_a, \text{ or } Q_l \times E \times C_a \qquad (13)$$

where CL_h = hepatic clearance (L/h), Q_l = blood flow rate to the metabolizing organ (L/h), and E = extraction ratio (i.e., organ clearance [L/h]/organ blood flow rate [L/h]).

Using Eq. 13, particularly, the form $Q_l{}^*E^*C_a$ instead of the conventional form (i.e., $V_{max}/K_m * C_{vl}$) to describe first-order metabolism in PBPK models is a starting point toward the exploration of animal-replacement approaches for simulating pharmacokinetics of chemicals. Before using $Q_l{}^*E^*C_a$ to simulate hepatic metabolism in PBPK models, it is essential to verify that this form and Michaelis-Menten equation-based form are mathematically equivalent. Recently, Poulin and Krishnan *(75)* have demonstrated the conceptual and mathematical equivalence of these two forms of equations. The determination of the equivalence was based on the fact that (1) $C_{vl} = C_a (1 - E)$, and (2) $V_{max}/K_m = Q_l{}^*E/(1 - E)$. The use of Eq. 13 permits to simulate the kinetics of chemicals with no knowledge of the actual numerical values of V_{max} and K_m, if the value of E can be specified. The E value, which represents the chemical-specific hepatic extraction ratio, or the magnitude of CL_h to Q_l cannot be obtained *a priori* at the present time without laboratory experimentation. Actually, V_{max} and K_m should be known in order to calculate the E values. However, it is common knowledge that for highly extracted chemicals, CL_h approximates Q_l, and for poorly extracted chemicals $CL_h \approx 0$. In other words, $E (= CL_h/Q_l)$ of chemicals range between 0 and 1. Therefore, by specifying $E = 0$ or 1 in Eq. 13 within PBPK models, predictions of the plausible envelope of tissue and blood concentration profiles can be generated for any inhaled VOC *(75)*. This methodology, which considers complete or zero hepatic extraction, can provide an envelope within which all experimental data should fall. Figures 4 and 5 present the predicted range of blood concentration profiles and their comparison with experimental data following inhalation exposure to 80 ppm of styrene in the rat and 100 ppm of dichloromethane in humans *(97,98)*. For generating these simulations, the E value in

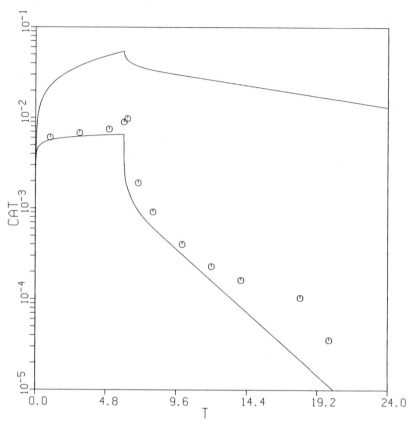

Fig. 4. Comparison of the PBPK model simulations (solid lines) of arterial blood concentration of styrene with experimental data (symbols) obtained in rats exposed to 80 ppm for 6 h. Simulations were obtained using tissue:air PCs and blood:air PCs predicted using Eqs. 3 and 9, and by setting E value to 0 (upper line) or 1 (lower line). The physiological parameters and PCs (oil:water and water:air) were obtained from Ramsey and Andersen *(97)* and Gargas et al. *(7)*. The data on rat tissue composition data were obtained from Table 2, whereas data on blood composition, concentration of binding proteins, and the association constant for hemoglobin binding were obtained from Poulin and Krishnan *(81)*.

the PBPK model was initially set equal to 0 and then to 1, and the PCs were predicted based on Eqs. 3, 4, and 9, respectively, in the human and rat PBPK models. This animal-replacement modeling approach is useful for VOCs with low $P_{b:a}$, since the ratio of the area-under-the-blood concentration vs time curves (AUC) obtained for conditions of $E = 0$ and $E = 1$ increases with increasing $P_{b:a}$ *(75)*.

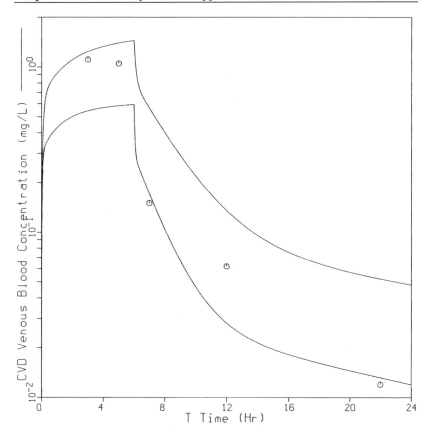

Fig. 5. Comparison of the PBPK model simulations (solid lines) of venous blood concentration of dichloromethane with experimental data (symbols) obtained in humans exposed to 100 ppm for 6 h. Simulations were obtained using tissue:air PCs and blood:air PCs predicted using Eqs. 3 and 4, and by setting E value to 0 (upper line) or 1 (lower line). The data sources for physiological parameters, human tissue and blood compositions, and PCs (oil:water and water:air) were Andersen et al. *(98)*, Poulin and Krishnan *(70)*, and Gargas et al. *(7)*, respectively.

Even though $AUC_{E=0/E=1}$ might be enormous in some cases, it only reflects the fact that this could actually happen in a population where the E value varies substantially, i.e., between 0 and 1 *(99)*. The use of the range of E values accounts not only for the interindividual differences in metabolism rates, but also for the possible effects of coexposures. Metabolic interactions during coexposures result in an increase or decrease of the extraction ratios; regardless of the mechanism, nature, and number of the interacting chemicals, the E value of a chemical will not exceed the range of 0 and 1. This animal-replacement approach can therefore be used to provide a first-cut estimation of the range of tissue doses and blood concentrations of chemicals that might result from specific exposure conditions. Further research to develop mechanism-based approaches for predicting animal-specific values and population distribution of the values of V_{max} and K_m is required. In this context, approaches based on thermodynamic principles *(100–103)* may be useful.

As detailed in this chapter, some progress has been made to develop mechanistic animal-replacement approaches for predicting pharmaco-kinetics of chemicals prior to animal or human experimentation. The applicability of these approaches has largely been verified with inhaled VOCs. Even though these approaches are conceptually applicable to nonvolatile organics as well, it becomes more challenging to predict the other PBPK model parameters required for modeling the kinetics of these chemicals (i.e., tissue diffusion coefficients, tissue binding as-sociation constants, oral absorption rates, and dermal permeability coefficients). As our level of understanding of the mechanistic deter-minants of each of these parameters improves, animal-replacement approaches to provide *a priori* predictions of these parameters can be developed. If similar strategies are explored for developing pharmacodynamic models as well, then animal-replacement approaches of modeling the toxicity of chemicals may become a realistic goal in the long run.

REFERENCES

1. Krishnan K, Andersen ME. Physiologically-based pharmacokinetic modeling in toxicology. In: Hayes W, ed. Principles and Methods in Toxicology, 3rd ed., Raven, New York, 1994, pp. 149–188.
2. Jain R, Gerlowski LE, Weissbrod JM, Wang J, Pierson RN. Kinetics of uptake, distribution and excretion of zinc in rats. Ann Biomed Eng 1982;9:347–361.
3. Bischoff KB, Dedrick RL, Zakharo DS, Longstreth JA. Methotrexate pharmaco-kinetics. J Pharm Sci 1971;60:1128–1133.
4. United States Environmental Protection Agency (USEPA), Dermal exposure assessment: principles and applications, Document EPA/600/8-91/011B, Office of health and environmental assessment, 1992.
5. Guengerich FP. *In vitro* techniques for studying metabolism. J Pharmacokinet Biopharm 1996;24:521–533.
6. Howes D, Guy RH, Hadgraft J, Heylings J, Hoeck U, Kemper F, et al. Methods for assessing percutaneous absorption. ATLA 1996;24:81–106.
7. Gargas ML, Burgess RJ, Voisard DE, Cason GH, Andersen ME. Partition coeffi-cients of low-molecular weight chemicals in various liquids and tissues. Toxicol Appl Pharmacol 1989;98:87–99.
8. Gargas ML, Seybold PG, Andersen ME. Modeling the tissues solubilities and metabolic rate constants (V_{max}) of halogenated methanes, ethanes, and ethylenes. Toxicol Lett 1988;43:235–256.

9. Fiserova-Bergerova V, Diaz ML. Determination and prediction of tissue-gas partition coefficients. Int Arch Occup Environ Health 1986;58:75–87.

10. Kaneko T, Wang PY, Sato A. Partition coefficients of some acetate esters and alcohols in water, blood, olive oil, and rat tissues. Occup Environ Med 1994; 54:68–72.

11. Connell Des W, Braddock RD, Mani SV. Prediction of the partition coefficient of lipophilic compounds in the air-mammal tissues systems. Sci Total Environ Suppl 1993;1383–1396.

12. Paterson S, Mackay D. Correlation of tissue, blood, and air partition coefficients of volatile organic chemicals. Br J Ind Med 1989;46:321–328.

13. Eger EI, Larson CP Jr. Anaesthetic solubility in blood and tissues; values and significance. Br J Anaesth 1964;36:140–149.

14. Lombardo F, Blake JF, Curatolo W. Computation of brain-blood partitioning of organic solutes via free energy calculations. J Med Chem 1996;39:4750–4755.

15. Abraham MH, Weathersby PK. Hydrogen bonding. 30. Solubility of gases and vapors in biological liquids and tissues. J Pharm Sci 1994;83:1450–1456.

16. Abraham MH, Kamlet MJ, Taft W, Doherty RM, Weathersby PK. Solubility properties in polymers and biological media: 2. The correlation and prediction of the solubilities of non electrolytes in biological tissues and fluids. J Med Chem 1985;28:865–870.

17. Morgan A, Black A, Belcher DR. Studies on the absorption of halogenated hydrocarbons and their excretions in breath using [38]Cl tracer techniques. Ann Occup Hyg 1972;15:273–282.

18. Cowle AL, Borgstedt HH, Gillies AJ. Solubilities of ethylene, cyclopropane, halothane and diethyl ether in human and dog blood at low concentrations. Anesthesiology 1971;35:203–211.

19. Feingold A. Estimation of anaesthetic solubility in blood. Anaesthesia Analgesia; Curr Res 1976;55:593–595.

20. Sato A, Nakajima T. Partition coefficients of some aromatic hydrocarbons and ketones in water, blood and oil. Br J Ind Med 1979;36:231–234.

21. Sato A, Nakajima T. A structure-activity relationship of some chlorinated hydrocarbons. Arch Environ Health 1979;34:69–75.

22. Pang YC, Reid PE, Brooks DE. Solubility and distribution of halothane in human blood. Br J Anaesthesia 1980;52:851–861.

23. Fiserova-Bergerova V, Tichy M, Di Carlo FJ. Effects of biosolubility on pulmonary uptake and disposition of gases and vapors of lipophilic chemicals. Drug Metab Rev 1984;15:1033–1070.

24. Tichy M, Fiserova-Bergerova V, Di Carlo FJ. QSAR. In: Tichy M, ed. Toxicology and xenobiochemistry, Elsevier Sciences Publishers, Amsterdam, 1984, pp. 225–231.

25. Tichy M. QSAR approach to estimation of the distribution of xenobiotics and the target organ in the body. Drug Metabol Drug Interact 1991;9:191–200.

26. Mattie DR, Bates GD Jr, Jepson GW, Fisher JW, McDougal JN. Determination of skin:air partition coefficients for volatile chemicals: experimental methods and applications. Fundam Appl Toxicol 1994;22:51–57.

27. Perbellini L, Brugnone F, Caretta D, Maranelli G. Partition coefficients of some industrial aliphatic hydrocarbons (C5-C7) in blood and human tissues. Br J Ind Med 1985;42:172–167.

28. Csanady GA, Laib RJ. Use of linear free energy relationships in toxicology: prediction of partition coefficients of volatile lipophilics compounds. Arch Toxicol 1990;64:594–596.

29. Yokogawa K, Nakashima E, Ishizaki J, Maeda H, Nagano T, Ichimura F. Relationships in the structure-tissue distribution of basic drugs in the rabbit. Pharm Res 1990;7:691–696.

30. Cabala R, Svobodova J, Felt L, Tichy M. Direct determination of partition coefficients of volatile liquids between oil and gas by gas chromatography and its use in QSAR analysis. Chromatographia 1992;34:601–606.

31. Parham FM, Mc Kohn MC, Matthews HB, De Rosa C, Portier CJ. Using structural information to create physiologically-based pharmacokinetic models for all polychlorinated biphenyls. Toxicol Appl Pharmacol 1997;144:340–347.

32. DeJongh J, Verhaar HJM, Hermes JLM. A Quantitative property relationship (QSPR) approach to estimate *in vitro* tissue:blood partition coefficients of organic chemicals in rats and humans. Arch Toxicol 1997;72:17–25.

33. Kalizan R, Markuszewski M. Brain/blood distribution described by a combination of partition coefficients and molecular mass. Int J Pharm 1996;145:9–16.

34. Steward A, Alott PR, Cowles AL, Mapleson WW. Solubility coefficients for inhaled anaesthetics for water, oil and biological media. Br J Anaesthesiol 1973;45:282–293.

35. Lerman J, Willis MM, Gregory GA, Eger EI. Osmolarity determines the solubility of anaesthetic in aqueous solutions at 37°C. Anaesthesiology 1973;59:554–559.

36. Scherertz EF, Sloan KB, McTiernan RG. Use of theoretical partition coefficients determined from solubility parameters to predict permeability coefficients for 5-fluorouracil. J Invest Dermatol 1987;89:147–151.

37. Brown SL, Rossi JE. A simple method for estimating dermal absorption of chemicals in water. Chemosphere 1989;19:1989–2001.

38. Tayar NE, Tsai RS, Testa B, Carrupt PA, Hansch C, Leo A. Percutaneous penetration of drugs: a quantitative structure-permeability relationship study. J Pharm Sci 1991;80:744–749.

39. McKone TE, Howe RA. Estimating dermal uptake of non ionic organic chemicals from water and soil: I. unified fugacity-based models for risk assessments. Risk Anal 1992;12:543–557.

40. Guy RH, Potts RO. Penetration of industrial chemicals across the skin: a predictive model. Am J Ind Med 1993;23:711–719.

41. Potts RO, Guy RH. Predicting skin permeability. Pharm Res 1992;9:663–669.

42. Potts RO, Guy RH. A predictive algorithm for skin permeability : the effects of molecular size and hydrogen bond activity. Pharm Res 1995;12:1628–1633.

43. Pugh WJ, Hadgraft J. Ab initio prediction of human skin permeability coefficients. Int J Pharm 1994;103:163–178.

44. Pugh WJ, Roberts MS, Hadgraft J. Epidermal permeability–penetrant structure relationships: 3. The effect of hydrogen bonding interactions and molecular size on diffusion across the stratum corneum. Int J Pharm 1996;138:149–165.

45. Roberts MS, Pugh WJ, Hadgraft J, Watkinson AC. Epidermal permeability-penetrant structure relationships: 1. An analysis of methods of predicting penetration of monofunctional solutes from aqueous solutions. Int J Pharm 1995;126: 219–233.

46. Roberts MS, Pugh WJ, Hadgraft J. Epidermal permeability: penetrant structure relationships: 2. The effect of H-bonding groups in penetrants on their diffusion through the stratum corneum. Int J Pharm 1996;132:23–32.

47. Bronaught RL, Barton CN. Prediction of human percutaneous absorption with physicochemical data. In: Wang RGM, Knaak JB, Maibach HI, eds. Risk Assessment. Dermal and Inhalation Exposure and Absorption of Toxicants. CRC, Boca Raton, 1993, pp. 117–126.

48. Maitani Y, Coutel-Egros A, Obata Y, Nagai T. Prediction of skin permeabilities of diclofenac and propanolol from theoretical partition coefficients determined from cohesion parameters. J Pharm Sci 1993;82:417–420.

49. Barratt MD. Quantitative structure-activity relationships for skin permeability. Toxicol In Vitro 1995;9:27–37.

50. Lien EJ, Gao H. QSAR analysis of skin permeability of various drugs in man as compared to *in vivo* and *in vitro* studies in rodents. Pharm Res 1995;12:583–587.

51. Wilshut A, ten Berge WF, Robinson PJ, McKone TE. Estimating skin permeation. The validation of five mathematical skin permeation models. Chemosphere 1995;30:1275–1296.

52. Kirchner LA, Moody RP, Doyle E, Boser JJ, Chu I. The prediction of skin permeability by using physicochemical data. ATLA 1997;25:359–370.

53. Cleek RL, Bunge AL. A new method for estimating dermal absorption from chemical exposure. 1. General approach. Pharm Res 1993;10:497–506.

54. Cnubben N, Peelen S, Borst JW, Vervoot J, Veeger C, Rietjens I. Molecular orbital-based quantitative structure-activity relationship for the cytochrome P450-catalysed 4-hydroxylation of halogenated anilines. Chem Res Toxicol 1994;7:590–598.

55. Cohen GM, Mannering GJ. Involvent of a hydrophobic site in the inhibition of the microsomal *p*-hydroxylation of aniline by alcohols. Mol Pharmacol 1973;9: 383–397.

56. Csanady Gy A, Laib RJ, Filser JG. Metabolic transformation of halogenated and other alkenes—a theoretical approach. Estimation of metabolic reactivities for *in vivo* conditions. Toxicol Lett 1995;75:217–223.

57. Ding T, van Rossum JM. K_s values of some homologous series of barbiturates and the relationship with the lipophilicity and metabolic clearance. Biochem Pharmacol 1977;26:2117–2130.

58. Waller CL, Evans MV, McKinney JD. Modeling the cytochrome P450-mediated metabolism of chlorinated volatile organic compounds. Drug Metab Dispos 1996;24:203–210.

59. Ishizaki J, Yokogawa K, Nakashima E, Ichimura F. Relationships between hepatic intrinsic clearance or blood cell-plasma partition coefficients in the rabbit and the lipophilicity of basic drugs. J Pharm Pharmacol 1997;49:768–772.

60. Straathof AJJ, Heijen JJ. Derivation of enzymatic rate equations using symbolic software. Biocatalysis Biotransformation 1997;15:29–37.

61. Szigeti L, Sevella B, Rezessy-Szabo J, Hoschke A. Estimation of the turnover number of laccase enxyme. Acta Alimentaria 1996;25:47–56.

62. Rietjens I, Soffers EMF, Hooiveld G, Veeger C, Vervoort J. Quantitative structure–activity relationships based on computer calculated parameters for the overall rate of gluthatione-*S*-transferase catalysed conjugation of a series of fluoronitrobenzenes. Chem Res Toxicol 1995;8:481–488.

63. Proost JH, Roggeveld J, Wierda J, Mark KH, Meijer Dirk KF. Relationship between chemical structure and physicochemical properties of series of bulky organic cations and their hepatic uptake and biliary excretion rates. J Pharmacol Exp Ther 1997;282:715–726.

64. Kim KH. 3D-Quantitative structure–activity relationships: describing hydrophobic interactions directly from 3D structures using a comparative molecular field analysis (CoMFA) approach. QSAR 1993;12:232–238.

65. Yamaguchi T, Yabuki M, Saito S, Watanabe T, Nishimura H, Isobe N, et al. Research to develop a predicting system of mammalian subacute toxicity (3) construction of a predictive toxicokinetics model. Chemosphere 1996;33:2441–2468.

66. Poorham FM, Portier CS. Using structural information to create physiologically-based pharmacokinetic models for all polychlorinated biphenyls. Toxicol Appl Pharmacol 1998;151:110–116.
67. Lowe HJ, Hagler K. Determination of volatile organic anaesthetic in blood, gases, tissues and lipids: partition coefficients. In: Porter R, ed. Gas Chromatography in Biology and Medicine. A Ciba-Geigy Foundation Symposium. Churchill, New York, 1969, pp. 86–103.
68. Falk A, Gullstrand E, Löf A, Wigaeus-Hjelm E. Liquid/air partition coefficients of four terpenes. Br J Ind Med 1990;47:62–64.
69. Poulin P, Krishnan K. A tissue composition-based algorithm for predicting tissue:air partition coefficients of organic chemicals. Toxicol Appl Pharmacol 1996;136:126–130.
70. Poulin P, Krishnan K. Molecular structure-based prediction of the partition coefficients of organic chemicals for physiological pharmacokinetic models. Toxicol Methods 1996;6:117–137.
71. Williams DP, Tung MA. Food dispersion. In: Fennema OR, Principles of Food Sciences, part I, Food Chemistry, Marcel Dekker, New York, 1976, pp. 530–575.
72. Poulin P, Krishnan K. A biologically-based algorithm for predicting human tissue:blood partition coefficients of organic chemicals. Hum Exp Toxicol 1995;14:273–280.
73. Klopman G, Ding C, Macina OT. Computer aided olive oil-gas partition coefficients calculations. J Chem Inf Comput Sci 1997;37:569–575.
74. Poulin P, Krishnan K. A Quantitative Structure-Toxicokinetic Relationship model for highly metabolized chemicals. ATLA 1998;26:45–49.
75. Poulin P, Krishnan K. Molecular structure-based prediction of the toxicokinetics of inhaled vapors in humans. Int J Toxicol, in press.
76. Pelekis M, Poulin P, Krishnan K. An approach for incorporating tissue composition data into physiologically-based pharmacokinetic models. Toxicol Ind Health 1995;11:511–522.
77. Poulin P, Krishnan K. An algorithm for predicting tissue:blood partition coefficients of organic chemicals from *n*-octanol:water partition coefficient data. J Toxicol Environ Health 1995;46:101–113.
78. Featherstone RM, Muehelbaecher CA, DeBon FL, Forsaith MS. Interaction of inert anaesthetic gases with proteins. Anaesthesiology 1961;22:977–981.
79. Larson CP Jr, Eger EI, Severinghaus JW. The solubility of halothane in blood and tissue homogenates. Anaesthesiology 1962;23:349–355.
80. Janberg J, Johanson G. Liquid/air partition coefficients of the trimethylbenzenes. Toxicol Ind Health 1995;11:81–88.
81. Poulin P, Krishnan K. A mechanistic algorithm for predicting blood:air partition coefficients of organic chemicals with the consideration of reversible binding in hemoglobin. Toxicol Appl Pharmacol 1996;136:131–137.
82. Johanson G, Dynésius B. Liquid/air partition coefficients of six commonly used glycol ethers. Br J Ind Med 1988;45:561–564.
83. Featherstone RM, Schoenborn BP. Protein and lipid binding of volatile anaesthetic agents. Br J Anaesthesiol 1964;36:150–154.
84. Lam CW, Gallen TJ, Boyd JF, Pierson DL. Mechanism of transport and distribution of organic solvents in blood. Toxicol Appl Pharmacol 1990;104:117–129.
85. Long B. Biochemist's Handbook. E & Spon, London, 1961.
86. Nelson GJ, ed. Lipid composition and metabolism of erythrocytes. In: Blood Lipids and Lipoproteins: Quantification, Composition and Metabolism. Wiley, New York, 1972, pp. 317–386.

87. Lentner C. Geigy Scientific Tables, vol. 3. Ciba-Geigy, New Jersey, 1981.
88. Johanson G, Nihlén A, Löf A. Toxicokinetics and acute effects of MTBE and ETBE in male volunteers. Toxicol Lett 1995;82/83:713–718.
89. Brown SH, Hattis D. The role of skin absorption as a route of exposure to volatile organic compounds in household tap water: a simulated approach. J Am Coll Toxicol 1989;8:839–851.
90. Shatkin JA, Brown HS. Pharmacokinetics of the dermal route of exposure to volatile organic chemicals in water; a computer simulation model. Environ Res 1991;56:90–98.
91. Nichols JW, McKlm M, Lien GJ, Hoffmann AD. Physiologically-based toxico-kinetic modeling of three waterborne chloroethanes in rainbow trout. Toxicol Appl Pharmacol 1991;110:374–389.
92. van Ommen B, deJongh J, van de Sandt J, Blaaudoer B, Hissink E, Bogaards J, et al. Computer-aided biokinetic modeling combined with in vitro data. Toxicol In Vitro 1995;9:537–542.
93. de Groot MJ, Kelder GM, Commandeur JNM, van Lenthe JH, Vermeulen NPE. Metabolites predictions for para-substituted anisoles based on ab initio complete active space self-consistent field calculations. Chem Res Toxicol 1995;8:437–443.
94. Koymans L, Vermeulen NPE, van Acker S, Koppele JM, Heykants JP, Lavrijsen K, et al. A predictive model for substrates of cytochrome P-450-debrisoquine (2D6). Chem Res Toxicol 1992;5:211–219.
95. Regan L, Bogle IDL, Dunnill P. Simulation and optimization of metabolic path-ways. Comput Chem Eng 1993;17:627–637.
96. Wilkinson GR, Shand DG. A physiological approach to hepatic drug clearance. Clin Pharmacol Ther 1975;18:377–390.
97. Ramsey JC, Andersen ME. A physiologically based description of the inhalation pharmacokinetics of styrene in rats and humans. Toxicol Appl Pharmacol 1984;73:159–175.
98. Andersen ME, Clewell HJ III, Gargas ML. Physiologically-based pharmacoki-netic modeling with dichloromethane, its metabolites carbon monoxide and blood carboxyhemoglobin in rats and humans. Toxicol Appl Pharmacol 1991;108:14–27.
99. Lavé Th, Dupin S, Schmitt C, Valles B, Ubeaud G, Chou RC, et al. The use of human hepatocytes to select compounds based on their expected hepatic extraction ratios in humans. Pharm Res 1997;14:152–155.
100. Akhrem AA, Metelitza DI, Bielski SM, Kiselev PA, Skurko ME, Usanov SA. Mechanism of oxygen activation in hydroxylation reactions involving cytochrome P-450. Croatica Chemica Acta 1977;49:223–235.
101. Akhrem AA, Bokut SB, Metelitza DI. The nature of the rate-limiting step in aniline hydroxylation involving cytochrome P-450 rat liver microsomes. Chem Biol Interact 1977;18:195–204.
102. Jung C, Ristau O. Mechanism of the cytochrome P-450 catalysed hydroxylation-thermodynamical aspects and the nature of the active oxygen species. Pharmazie 1978;33:329–331.
103. Chan Z, Hollobone BR. A QSAR for steroidal compound interaction with cyto-chrome P 4501A1. Environ Toxicol Chem 1995;14:597–603.

IV Use of Alternatives
in Hazard Assessment Initiatives

12 Validation of the Cytosensor™ Microphysiometer for In Vitro Cytotoxicity Testing

R. J. Mioduszewski, PhD, C. J. Cao, MD, PhD, M. E. Eldefrawi, PhD, A. T. Eldefrawi, PhD, D. E. Menking, MS, and J. J. Valdes, PhD

Contents

INTRODUCTION
METHODS
RESULTS
DISCUSSION
CONCLUSIONS
ACKNOWLEDGMENTS
REFERENCES

INTRODUCTION

Regulatory agencies addressing human risk assessment of new pharmaceuticals, pesticides, food additives, cosmetics, and other chemicals currently require submission of a large battery of in vivo toxicity data derived from tests utilizing laboratory animals. Although fairly well proven for evaluating toxicity, the use of laboratory animals may have limited predictive values for human risk assessment because of differences in factors, such as bioavailability, pharmacokinetics, metabolism, receptor sensitivity, and repair mechanisms. The use of cell cultures for measuring drug toxicity is becoming increasingly acceptable. Accordingly, in vitro toxicity tests have been in demand and numerous organizations

From: *Toxicity Assessment Alternatives: Methods, Issues, Opportunities*
Edited by: H. Salem and S. A. Katz © Humana Press Inc., Totowa, NJ

(e.g., Fund for Replacement of Animals in Medical Experiments [FRAME], European Research Group for Alternate Testing [ERGAT], Center for Alternatives to Animal Testing [CAAT], and the International Multi-Center Evaluation of In Vitro Cytotoxicity [MEIC]) are encouraging the development of alternative testing protocols.

The in vitro toxicity studies described below utilize the Cytosensor™*, a silicon-based microphysiometer, designed to measure changes in the metabolic rates of living cells by monitoring the rate at which cells excrete acidic metabolic products *(1–4)*. It has been used to monitor the response of cells to ligands of ionotropic, metabolic, and tyrosine kinase receptors *(3)*, the response to skin and ocular irritants *(5)*, to cytokines *(6)*, and to antineoplastic agents *(1)*.

Although hundreds of in vitro assays of general toxicity have been proposed, in order to establish in vitro methods as supplements or alternatives to animal tests, they must be validated. The most important determinants of in vitro assay validity should be a functional relationship with, and the predictive characteristics relative to, the intended in vivo response. One such initiative was undertaken by the MEIC. This project has been organized by the Scandinavian Society of Cell Toxicology and involves a number of laboratories from different countries. The initial thrust of this exercise has been the toxicological assessment of a list of up to 50 chemicals by a wide variety of alternative techniques and a subsequent analysis of the predictability of these tests against in vivo data.

The present studies were intended as "prevalidation" experiments to characterize the effects of different exposure protocols and human cell types for basal cytotoxicity applications involving the Cytosensor™ microphysiometer. Because potential toxicants primarily affect select target organs, specific cell lines (e.g., neuronal and liver) were tested to identify characteristics of organ-specific toxicity.

METHODS

Test Chemicals

Acetaminophen, acetylsalicylic acid, ferrous sulfate, diazepam, amitriptyline, and digoxin were obtained from Sigma Chemical Co. (St. Louis, MO). Ethanol was obtained from a local supplier. Ethylene glycol, methanol, and isopropanol were obtained from Baker Chemical Co. (Phillipsburg, NJ). These 10 drugs are identified as the first 10 MEIC chemicals.

*Cytosensor™ is a registered trademark symbol of Molecular Devices Corporation, Inc., Sunnyvale, CA.

Cell Culture and Maintenance

The human liver cell line (ATCC CCL-13), a nonmalignant cell line established in 1954, and a human neuroblastoma line, SK-N-SH (ATCC HTB-11), were obtained from the American Type Culture Collection (Manassas, VA). The cells were grown in the recommended basal medium Eagle (BME) culture medium with Earle's BSS 90%, calf serum 10% at 37°C and at 5% CO_2 atmosphere. Subcultures were prepared weekly using a 1:4 subcultivation ratio.

Measurement of Cellular Metabolic Rates

Human liver cells were harvested from culture flasks and plated into sterile specially designed cell capsule cups (Molecular Devices Corp., Sunnyvale, CA) at a density of 2×10^5 cells/mL/cup. Likewise, in separate experiments, human neuroblastoma cells were plated at a density of $1–3 \times 10^5$ cells/mL/cup. Within 1 d of preparation, the seeded cups were placed into their microvolume flow chambers in the Cytosensor™ and low buffering capacity Minimum Essential Medium (MEM) from Gibco-BRL (Rockville, MD) that contained 5 mM glucose, was pumped at 0.1 mL/min through the chambers.

Protocols for Exposure of Human Cells to Test Chemicals

Two protocols were used to collect data on the response of human liver or neuronal cell lines to drugs: the first was a long-term (24-h) exposure protocol (used only on the human liver cell line), in which cells were exposed to the drug for 20 h, while plated in the capsule cups. Exposure to the drug continued for an additional 4 h in the Cytosensor by adding the drug at the same concentration to the perfusing assay MEM medium. The cells were then perfused with drug-free MEM medium for 1 h. Untreated controls were included in each run and used to determine the basal metabolic activity for each particular passage of the human liver cells. The rate of acidification (μV/s) during this protocol was recorded every 6 min.

To select the concentration range for testing, four concentrations for each drug, ranging from 100-fold lower to 100-fold higher than the published concentrations that induce any of a variety of morphological/metabolic changes compromising cell homeostasis or viability in 50% of the exposed cell population (IC_{50}), were used. Based on the results of these bracketing tests, three concentrations that would inhibit metabolic activity to between 10 and 90% were selected for each drug and used to generate concentration–effect relationships from which IC_{50} values were determined. In this protocol, control levels were established on a different population of cells that was part of the same harvest, but had never been exposed to any of the drugs. In a typical experiment of 4- or 24-h duration, two channels were used for controls and six channels were used for testing chemicals. Values of untreated (control) and treated cells at the end of the 24 h were used to calculate the percent inhibition of metabolic activity induced by each chemical at the indicated concentration.

The second protocol (used in both liver and neuroblastoma cell lines) was a 4-h exposure, where the basal metabolic activity in all channels was recorded during the first hour prior to the introduction of the MEIC chemical, so that the same population of cells served as its own control. The test chemical was added to the MEM medium 1 h after the basal acidification rate was established. Starting with the lowest concentration, the effects on acidification rates were monitored once every 2 min for 30 min. This step was repeated using the next highest concentration until five concentrations were tested for each chemical. Reversibility of the chemical effect was monitored during the final stage of exposure to chemical-free medium.

Data Acquisition and Analysis

Extracellular levels of acidification (pH or μV) were recorded and plotted as a function of time and reported every second to the computer. For measurement of metabolic rate, the flow of medium was halted for 30 s. During this period, the cells would acidify the medium in the chamber at the surface of the silicon sensor. The metabolic rate was measured as the slope of a linear least-square fit of the extracellular pH (or μV) vs time data, while flow was interrupted. The percent of irreversible change in metabolic rate was used as an index of cell death. Acidification rates were monitored continuously by the computer and printed out as raw values (μV/s) or as percent change from control. The latter established the control acidification rate as 100 and recorded changes as % of control. The median inhibitory concentration (IC_{50}) to cellular acidification rate for each test chemical was obtained as a mean $\pm$ SEM from semilogarithmic plots of the results of three experiments.

RESULTS

The IC_{50} values for the 10 MEIC chemicals tested were approx 10-fold higher under the short-exposure protocol conditions than results obtained with the 24-h exposure protocol in human liver cells (Table 1).

In human liver cells, the alcohols, ethanol, methanol and isopropanol enhanced metabolic activity in a concentration-dependent manner in the short exposure protocol, but decreased it in the 24-h exposure protocol.

Table 1
Average Toxic Concentrations of MEIC Chemicals (#1–10): In Vivo Human Lethal Plasma Concentrations vs In Vitro Indices of Human Cytotoxicity (IC_{50})

MEIC chemical	In vivo, mM — Human[a] lethal plasma concentration	In vitro, human cell lines, IC_{50}, mM — Cytosensor, liver—24 h	Cytosensor, liver—4 h	Cytosensor, neuroblastoma—4 h	$MTT^{b,c}$, liver—24 h
Paracetamol	9.9	9.4	60	21.6	6.6
Acetylsalicylic acid	3.6	10.3	100	9.7	4.97
Ferrous sulfate	0.340	0.6	5.0	0.4	6.4
Diazepam	0.250	0.59	4.0	1.3	0.23
Amitriptyline	0.054	0.05	0.5	0.6	0.054
Digoxin	0.00003	0.0009	0.3	0.13	0.0000049
Ethylene glycol	48.0	291.7	>800	910.0	138.0
Methanol	60.0	195.0	>800	465.0	819.0
Ethanol	150.0	107.8	>800	351.0	303.0
Isopropanol	67.0	73.2	>600	223.0	125.0

[a]Data from (7).

[b]Data from (8), performed in human hepatocytes.

[c]MTT is a methylthiazol tetrazolium dye, which is taken up into the cells and converted from a soluble yellow-colored chemical to a blue precipitate indicative of mitochondrial functional integrity and cell viability.

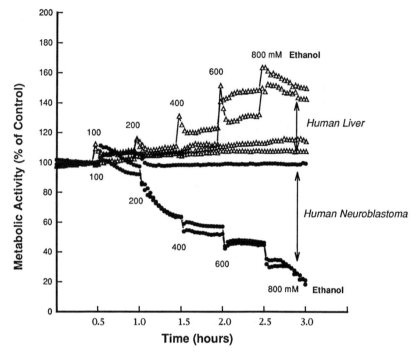

Fig. 1. Effects of ethanol exposure (4 h) on metabolic activity in liver versus neuronal human cell lines.

In contrast, metabolic activity was inhibited by the above alcohols in human neuroblastoma cells under the short protocol. The ethanol data are used for illustration of results obtained with the short protocol (Fig. 1). Ethylene glycol at 100–800 m*M* inhibited metabolic activity in human liver cells. However, the degree of inhibition was so small that at 800 m*M*, only 40% inhibition was achieved in the short protocol.

Published values of human lethal blood concentrations (Table 1) collected by the Swedish Poison Information Center, Stockholm have been used *(7)* for correlation with in vitro cytotoxicity data. These same lethal blood concentrations were used to correlate the cytotoxicity of the first 10 MEIC chemicals obtained with the Cytosensor™, including their toxicities in human liver cells measured under the long- (24-h) (Fig. 2), and short- (4-h) (Fig. 3) exposure protocols in liver and the short protocol in neuroblastoma cells (Fig. 4). Cytotoxicity measured after 24 h of exposure in human liver cells correlated highly with human toxic blood concentrations (*r* = 0.97). On the other hand, cytotoxicity measured by the short-exposure protocol could be assessed for only the first six chemicals in liver cells. Ethyl, methyl, and isopropyl alcohols (MEIC

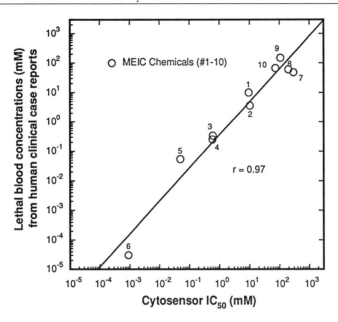

Fig. 2. Toxicity of MEIC chemicals (#1–10): in vitro (human liver cells, IC_{50}, 24-h exposure) vs in vivo human lethal blood concentrations.

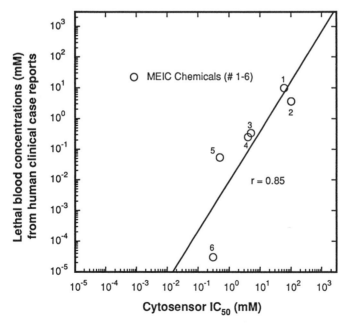

Fig. 3. Toxicity of MEIC chemicals (#1–10): in vitro (human liver cells, IC_{50}, 4-h exposure) vs in vivo human lethal blood concentrations.

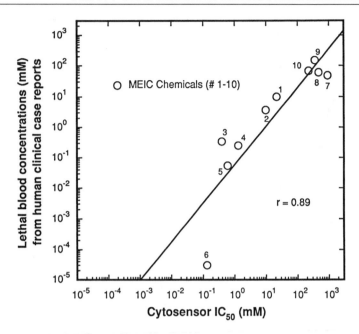

Fig. 4. Toxicity of MEIC chemicals (#1–10): in vitro (human neuroblastoma cells, IC_{50}, 4-h exposure) vs in vivo human lethal blood concentrations.

chemicals no. 8–10) in Table 1 and ethylene glycol (no. 7) inhibited acidification rates in liver cells at concentrations higher than 400 mM, but failed to inhibit 50% of the control levels at the highest concentrations tested in liver cells. Accordingly, no IC_{50} values were obtained (Table 1), and they were excluded from the plot correlating cytotoxicity to human lethal blood concentrations ($r = 0.85$) (Fig. 3). In contrast, all chemicals inhibited acidification rates of neuroblastoma cells during the short protocol with a significant correlation of IC_{50} values with human lethal blood concentrations ($r = 0.89$) (Fig. 4). Although not shown in Figs. 3 or 4, there appeared to be better correlation between IC_{50} values and human lethal blood concentrations when the digoxin data were excluded ($r = 0.96$, liver, short exposure protocol, and $r = 0.96$, neuroblastoma cells). Such differences were not noted using the 24-h exposure protocol in liver cells and may involve basal cytotoxic mechanisms, which require a longer exposure time for expression.

DISCUSSION

These data demonstrate that monitoring cellular metabolic activity of human cell lines is a reproducible, and accurate yet nonspecific index of cytotoxicity for estimating the relative exposure hazards of chemicals in humans. Chemical-induced reduction in cellular acidification rate monitored by the Cytosensor™ is likely the result of some combination of a lowered number of viable cells (i.e., an irreversible effect shown after washing the chemical from the perfusion media) and a lowered metabolic rate reflecting cellular damage on a permanent or temporary basis throughout the exposed cell population.

Both the magnitude and kinetics of the cell response to chemical exposure depend on a variety of factors that include type and activity of cell receptors in addition to the chemical's concentration and duration of exposure. Duration of toxicant exposure is a determining factor in not only the severity of a cytotoxic response, but also its onset and duration. For example, ethanol (100 mM) enhanced metabolic rate of liver cells during the brief 30-min exposure period in the 4-h exposure protocol, whereas metabolic rate was irreversibly inhibited in liver cells after 24 h of exposure to the same concentration. It is obvious that the cells receiving the 24-h exposure of ethanol received a much greater dosage, thus resulting in irreversible metabolic inhibition. This may be explained, in part, by the removal of toxic metabolites by the perfusion media in the Cytosensor™, which is more similar to in vivo conditions, but contrary to other in vitro assay conditions which involve a static exposure. Nevertheless, the 24-h exposure data correlate better than the 4-h data with published human toxic blood concentrations. Longer exposure time (i.e., 72 h) was found to be even more suitable for the assessment of potential toxicity by two in vitro cytotoxicity tests than the 24-h exposure, which is less likely to allow sufficient time for certain chemicals to exert their toxic effects, particularly for chemicals that inhibit cell division or affect cell viability through other long-term effects *(9)*. On the other hand, the 4-h exposure protocol allows more rapid screening of chemicals.

It is interesting that even under conditions of identical concentration and exposure duration, a chemical, such as ethanol (Fig. 1), may have opposite effects on cellular metabolic rate, depending on the type of cell line involved. These findings suggest that a response to certain chemicals is in part determined by cellular features of a particular target organ in addition to a general cytotoxic response. In addition, they also suggest the potential utility of a battery of cell types vs a single cell type in cytotoxicity screening for the purpose of estimating human health hazards of chemical exposure.

A variety of end points have been used in in vitro toxicology studies, including changes in cell morphology, viability (e.g., trypan blue exclusion, neutral red uptake, or MTT colormetric assay), adhesion, cell proliferation (DNA or RNA increase), membrane damage (loss of enzymes, e.g., lactate dehydrogenase; LDH), uptake of radioactive precursors, and metabolic effects (e.g., impairment of mitochondrial function) *(10)*. The present Cytosensor™ data correlate well not only with human lethal plasma concentration data (Figs. 1–3), but also with other in vitro data as represented by the MTT uptake assay data of Jover et al. *(8)* (Table 1). For some of the MEIC compounds tested here, the cytosensor appeared to detect signs of basal cytotoxicity at lower concentrations as compared to the MTT assay (Table 1).

Ideally, the in vitro test system should match the in vivo target in terms of differentiated properties, including metabolic capacity, and surface and intracellular receptors that are target molecules *(10)*. On the other hand, general or basal cytotoxicity involves fundamental structures and functions common to all cells (e.g., cell membrane integrity, protein or DNA synthesis, mitochondrial function). Basal cytotoxicity data are highly reproducible and show a good correlation with intrinsic toxic potencies measured in vivo *(11,12)* and provide a baseline for interpretation of results obtained in target organ toxicity studies.

It may be essential to conduct basal cytotoxicity alongside target organ cytotoxicity, a comparison that can be achieved by the Cytosensor™. For example, using a short-exposure protocol, the effect of a chemical on cells from eight different organs (e.g. liver, kidney, skin, brain, and so forth) can be determined in a single experiment. The most sensitive cell type that is affected by the lowest drug concentration in the shortest time will be identified as possibly the primary cell target for that drug; for example, hepatocytes would be more sensitive to hepatotoxic chemicals and neuronal cells to neurotoxic chemicals. The data presented above suggested that ethanol is a more potent neurotoxicant than a hepatotoxicant. Basal cytotoxicity is often characterized as involving long-term (i.e., hours) effects and, thus, may not be as relevant to neurotoxic drugs, most of which may produce their effects in minutes. Organ-specific testing would be more relevant. An example is the identification of end points in human neuroblastoma cells that are altered by neurotoxicants at 100- to 1000-fold lower concentrations than those affecting cell viability.

CONCLUSIONS

A unique feature of the Cytosensor™ microphysiometer is its ability to monitor cellular metabolic effects of test chemical exposure conditions continuously (including concentration and duration) as well as their reversibility. Good correlations were found between indices of basal cytotoxic effects (IC_{50}) of the first 10 MEIC chemicals on human liver and neuronal cells with reported lethal concentrations in human blood. However, metabolic responses to chemical exposure may be dependent on cell type and exposure conditions. Application of the Cytosensor™ to studies of in vitro basal cytotoxicity using human cell lines could provide a rapid screen for estimating acute health hazards in humans.

ACKNOWLEDGMENTS

This research was supported by the US Army Edgewood Research, Development and Engineering Center, APG, MD 21010-5423.

REFERENCES

1. Parce JW, Owicki JC, Kercso KM. Detection of cell affecting agents with a silicon biosensor. Science 1989;246, 243–247.
2. Parce JW, Owicki JC, Wada HG, Kercso KM. Cells on silicon: the microphysiometer: In: Goldberg AM, ed. In Vitro Toxicology: Mechanisms and New Technology. Mary Ann Liebert, New York, 1991, pp. 97–106.
3. Owicki JC, Parce JW, Kersco KM, Sigal GB, Muir VC, Venter JC, et al. Continuous monitoring of receptor-mediated changes in the metabolic rates of living cells. Proc Natl Acad Sci USA 1990;87:4007–4011.
4. Owicki JC, Parce JW. Biosensors based on the energy metabolism of living cells: The physical chemistry and cell biology of extracellular acidification. Biosensors Bioelectronics 1992;7:255–272.
5. Bruner LH, Miller KR, Owicki JC, Parce JW, Muir VC. Testing ocular irritancy in vitro with the silicon microphysiometer. Toxicol In Vitro 1991;5:277–284.
6. McConnell HM, Owicki JC, Parce JW, Miller DL, Baxter GT, Wada HG, et al. The cytosensor microphysiometer: Biological applications of silicon technology. Science 1992;257:1906–1912.
7. Eckwall B, Bondesson I, Castell JV, Gomez-Lechon MJ, Hellberg S, Hogberg J, et al. Cytotoxicity evaluation of the first ten MEIC chemicals: acute lethal toxicity in man predicted by cytotoxicity in five cellular assays and oral LD_{50} tests in rodents. ATLA 1989;17:83–100.
8. Jover R, Ponsoda X, Castell JV, Gomez-Lechon MJ. Evaluation of cytotoxicity of ten chemicals on human cultured hepatocytes: predictability of human toxicity and comparison with rodent culture system. Toxicol In Vitro 1992;6:47–52.
9. Riddell RJ, Panacer DS, Wilde SM, Clothier RH, Ball, M. The importance of exposure period and cell type: in vitro cytotoxicity tests. ATLA 1986;14:86–92.
10. Balls M, Fenton JH. The use of basal cytotoxicity and target organ toxicity tests in hazard identification and risk assessment. ATLA 1992;20:368–388.
11. Clothier RH, Hulme LM, Smith M, Balls M. Comparison of the in vitro cytotoxicities and acute in vivo toxicities of 59 chemicals. Mol Toxicol 1987;1:571–577.
12. Fry JR, Garle MJ, Hammond AH. Choice of acute toxicity measures for comparison of in vivo-in vitro toxicity. ATLA 1988;16:175–179.

13 Sulfur Mustard Effects on Cell Yield Alter Viability Assessment in Normal Human Epidermal Keratinocytes

Janet Moser, DVM, PhD, Susan A. Kelly, BS, and Henry L. Meier, PhD

CONTENTS

INTRODUCTION

Sulfur mustard (HD; 2,2'-dichlorodiethyl sulfide) is a vesicant chemical warfare agent that produces injuries to the skin, eyes, and lungs. It has been a military threat since its first use as a chemical warfare agent during World War I. To develop antivesicant therapeutic regimens, adult human peripheral blood lymphocytes (PBL) and normal human eqidermal keratinocytes (NHEK) have been used as models to study the cytotoxic effects of HD. Following HD exposure to the cells, changes in cellular biochemical markers, such as adenosine triphosphate (ATP), nicotinamide adenine dinucleotide (NAD), DNA, proteases, and viability have been studied. Previous investigations have demonstrated that cell viability decreases when NHEK *(1–3)* and PBL *(2–4)* are exposed to increasing concentrations of HD. It has also been reported that NHEK

From: *Toxicity Assessment Alternatives: Methods, Issues, Opportunities*
Edited by: H. Salem and S. A. Katz © Humana Press Inc., Totowa, NJ

155

are more resistant than PBL to the cytotoxic effects of HD *(2)*. These studies, however, did not take into consideration cell recovery. Time and concentration effects of HD on cell yield (number of cells recovered) have not been reported. While investigating HD-dependent DNA changes in NHEK and PBL, we observed a substantial difference in the cytotoxic effects of HD on NHEK from what was previously reported *(2)*. To elucidate the discrepancy between our findings and previously published work, the effects of HD on viability, as defined by propidium iodide exclusion, and cell yield were studied.

MATERIALS AND METHODS

Primary cultures of adult NHEK were obtained from Clonetics Corporation, San Diego, CA. Tertiary cultures of NHEK were passed into 75-cm^2 tissue-culture flasks or six-well plates and grown until 50–70% confluent. They were then exposed to various concentrations of HD (0.01–1.0 m*M*) and harvested at various times after exposure (up to 24 h). Viability was assessed by propidium iodide exclusion *(2)* using a FACSort flow cytometer (Becton Dickinson, San Jose, CA, USA). The data were analyzed with the Lysis II computer software program (Becton Dickinson). Cells were counted using the Coulter Counter, Model ZM (Coulter Electronics Limited, Luton, Beds., England). To observe cell fragments microscopically, samples were stained with trypan blue dye and viewed by light microscopy.

To obtain fresh human PBL, blood was drawn by venipuncture from normal human volunteers under an approved human use protocol. The PBL were isolated from blood by centrifugation using a Percoll gradient (density = 1.080 g/mL at 20°C) as previously described *(5)*. The PBL were plated into 24-well plates, exposed to various concentrations of HD (0.01 to 1.0 m*M*), and harvested at selected times after exposure (up to 24 h). Lymphocyte viability and yield were determined as performed for NHEK. All experiments were conducted at least in triplicate with similar results.

RESULTS

Percent viability decreased with increasing concentration of HD in both NHEK and PBL 24 h after HD exposure (Fig. 1A,B, respectively). The HD concentration that produced the highest loss in viability (greatest amount of propidium iodide incorporation) in NHEK was 0.6 m*M* and in PBL, 0.3 m*M*. At low concentrations, percent viability decreased to a greater extent in PBL than in NHEK as HD concentration increased.

Twenty-four hours after HD exposure, there was a loss in NHEK yield between 0.06 and 1.0 m*M* HD (Fig. 2A). The decrease in NHEK

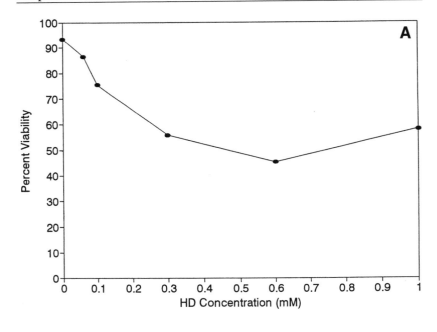

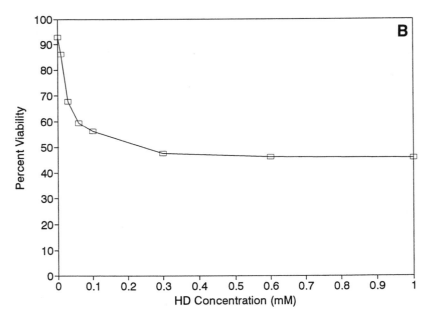

Fig. 1. (A,B) The effect of HD concentration on NHEK **(A)** and PBL **(B)** viability. Cells were exposed to buffer or to buffer plus the indicated HD concentrations, and harvested 24 h after exposure. Viability was measured by propidium iodide exclusion with flow cytometry.

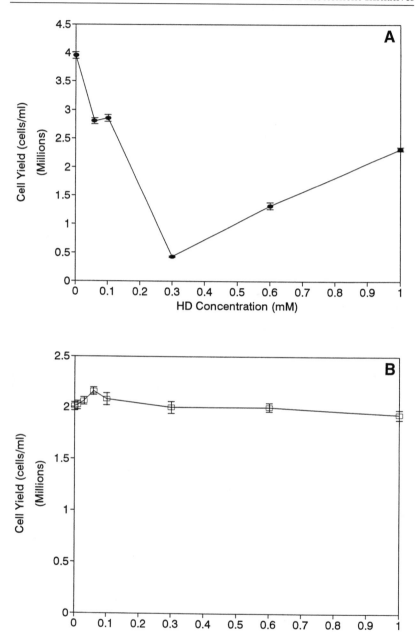

Fig. 2. (A,B) The effect of HD concentration on NHEK **(A)** and PBL **(B)** yield. Cells were exposed to buffer or to buffer plus the indicated HD concentrations, harvested 24 h after exposure, and counted in quadruplicate on a Coulter counter. Data are mean ± 1 SD of cell yield.

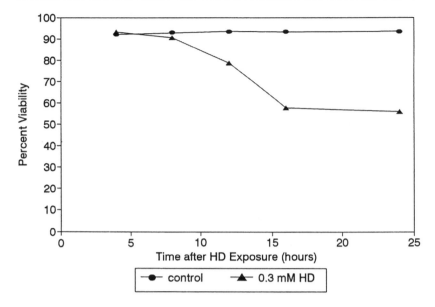

Fig. 3. A time-dependent decrease in NHEK viability after HD exposure. Cells were exposed to buffer (control) or to buffer plus 0.3 mM HD, and were harvested at the times indicated. Viability was assessed by propidium iodide exclusion with flow cytometry.

yield was associated with an increase in trypan blue-stained fragments observed on slides. The HD concentration that produced the lowest NHEK yield was 0.3 mM. The maximum loss in NHEK yield did not always occur at the same HD concentration as the maximum loss in NHEK viability. The PBL yield remained constant throughout the HD concentration range (Fig. 2B). The extensive formation of trypan blue-stained fragments was not detected in PBL exposed to the same concentrations of HD as NHEK.

Propidium iodide incorporation in NHEK increased with time following HD exposure; after exposure to 0.3 mM HD, propidium iodide incorporation began to occur after a 4-h latent period (Fig. 3). In PBL, propidium iodide incorporation increased with increasing HD concentration and began, as with NHEK, 4 h after HD exposure (data not shown).

Between 8 and 12 h, the number of control NHEK began to increase, and they nearly doubled in 24 h (Fig. 4). However, the number of NHEK exposed to 0.3 mM HD did not increase over time and began to decrease between 12 and 16 h. The NHEK yield was <1/10 that of control cells 24 h after exposure. There was no change in PBL yield over the entire time-course (data not shown).

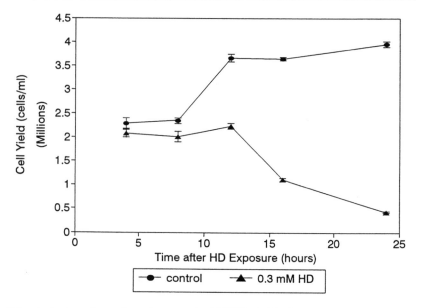

Fig. 4. A time-dependent decrease in NHEK yield after HD exposure. Cells were exposed to buffer (control) or to buffer plus 0.3 m*M* HD, and were harvested at the times indicated. Cells were counted in quadruplicate on a Coulter counter. Data are mean ± 1 SD of NHEK yield.

The NHEK were at least twice as sensitive as PBL to HD-induced cytotoxicity, and by 24 h, viable NHEK yield was only 6% in those cells exposed to 0.3 m*M* HD (Fig. 5A). In PBL, there was an HD concentration and time-dependent loss in percent viable yield; percent viable yield decreased to 60% 18 h after exposure to 0.1 and 0.6 m*M* HD (Fig. 5B). In the PBL, exposure to 0.01 m*M* HD produced no loss in percent viable yield (overlaps the control).

In PBL, there was almost a linear decrease in percent viable yield from 0.01 to 1.0 m*M* HD (log scale; Fig. 6). In NHEK, there was a decrease in percent viable yield that appeared to follow a sigmoid curve with a moderate decrease at low HD concentrations and a sharp decrease between 0.1 and 0.3 m*M* HD (log scale). The NHEK were more susceptible to HD-induced cytotoxicity than PBL.

DISCUSSION

Both adult NHEK and human PBL exposed to HD demonstrate an HD concentration and time-dependent loss in viability. However, only adult NHEK exposed to HD demonstrate an HD concentration and time-

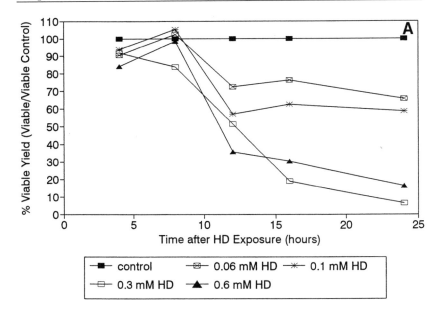

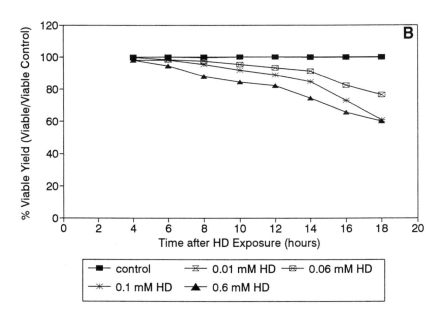

Fig. 5. (A,B) A time-dependent decrease in viable NHEK (**A**) and PBL (**B**) yield after HD exposure. Cells were exposed to buffer (control) or to buffer plus the indicated HD concentrations, and were harvested at the times indicated. Percent viable yield was obtained by dividing the number of viable cells in each sample by the number of viable control cells.

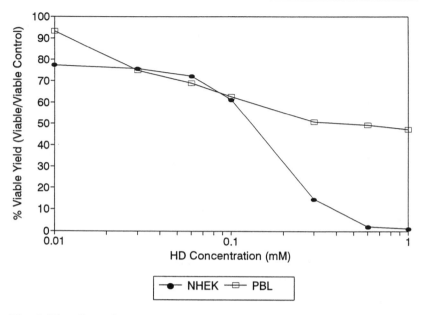

Fig. 6. The effect of HD concentration on viable NHEK and PBL yield. Cells were exposed to buffer plus the indicated HD concentrations, harvested 24 h after exposure, and percent viable yield determined as for Fig. 5. Data are graphed on a log scale.

dependent loss in cell yield. Loss in NHEK yield appears to be the result of NHEK fragmentation produced by HD. Human PBL exposed to HD demonstrate no loss in cell yield as a function of HD concentration or time after exposure.

Fragmented dead NHEK are not included in the total cell count when percent viability is determined. Therefore, cytotoxicity of HD is almost certainly greater than that reflected in percent viability alone. Taking into account both viability and cell yield, NHEK appear to be more susceptible to HD-induced cytotoxicity than PBL, contrary to previously published conclusions *(2)*.

Both NHEK yield and viability must be considered when interpreting results of studies that involve cellular biochemical changes that are induced by HD. Results of previous studies into HD effects on cellular biochemical markers and HD cytotoxic mechanisms in NHEK may need to be re-evaluated. Actual viable cell counts, rather than percent viability alone (as measured by dye exclusion), should be taken into account when using any cellular model to study cytotoxic mechanisms.

REFERENCES

1. Smith WJ, Gross CL, Chan P, Meier HL. The use of human epidermal keratinocytes in culture as a model for studying the biochemical mechanisms of sulfur mustard toxicity. Cell Biol Toxicol 1990;6:285–291.

2. Smith WJ, Sanders KM, Gales YA, Gross CL. Flow cytometric analysis of toxicity by vesicating agents in human cells in vitro. J Toxicol Cutan Occu Toxicol 1991;10:33–42.

3. Smith WJ, Sanders KM, Caulfield JE, Gross CL. Sulfur mustard-induced biochemical alterations in proliferating human cells in culture. J Toxicol Cutan Occu Toxicol 1992;11:293–304.

4. Meier HL, Johnson JB. Inhibitors of poly(ADP-ribose) polymerase prevent the cytotoxic effects induced in human lymphocytes by the alkylating agent, 2,2'-dichlorodiethyl sulfide (sulfur mustard, HD). Toxicol App Pharm 1992;113: 234–239.

5. Meier HL, Gross CL, Papirmeister B. 2,2'-dichlorodiethyl sulfide (sulfur mustard) decreases NAD$^+$ levels in human leukocytes. Toxicol Lett 1987;39:109–122.

14 Development of Human Keratinocyte Colonies for Confocal Microscopy and for Study of Calcium Effects on Growth Differentiation and Sulfur Mustard Lesions

A Model

Robert J. Werrlein, PhD,
Tracey A. Hamilton,
and Janna S. Madren-Whalley

Contents

INTRODUCTION

One of the most fascinating questions about sulfur mustard (HD) injuries is the unanswered issue of why basal cells are specific targets for vesicating lesions. What mechanism sets basal cells apart from all other cells of the epidermis and causes their interface with the basement membrane to be the primary site for blister formation? In recent studies with confocal microscopy, Werrlein et al. *(1)* reported that increased extracellular calcium affected the morphology and in vitro response of

From: *Toxicity Assessment Alternatives: Methods, Issues, Opportunities*
Edited by: H. Salem and S. A. Katz © Humana Press Inc., Totowa, NJ

human epidermal keratinocytes (HEK) to HD. The image changes observed were consistent with discoveries by Hennings et al. *(2–4)* that small increases in extracellular calcium (as little as 0.01 mM) can cause fast-acting, dramatic responses in the differentiation of keratinocytes. Kruszewski et al. *(5)* demonstrated that keratinocytes can respond to small incremental calcium changes (of 0.1–0.12 mM) within 60 s, but noted that the capacity for transient response to calcium was lost as keratinocytes differentiated. Others have demonstrated that calcium-induced terminal differentiation can alter cell-surface receptors *(6)* and epidermal protein markers *(7,8)*. Complementary studies *(9–11)* have demonstrated that calcium gradients exist in the epidermis of mice and humans, with the lowest calcium concentrations residing at the basal layer. Each has determined that basal cells exist in an environment that is relatively low in calcium when compared to keratinocytes located in the suprabasal layers of the epidermis. Absolute calcium concentrations within the gradient have not been determined. It is known, however, that epidermal gradients can be disrupted by certain chemicals, e.g., acetone and lovastatin *(12)*, by diseases like psoriasis *(13,14)*, and by essential fatty acid deficiencies *(12)*. Based on the evidence accumulated, we have proposed that exposure to HD may disrupt extracellular calcium gradients or programmed responses to calcium, which would be especially disruptive to basal cells because they are more sensitive to changes in calcium concentration than are differentiated keratinocytes. To test this hypothesis, we have initiated development of primary and first-passage keratinocyte cultures from human skin resections that will allow us to use confocal microscopy to determine how calcium concentration affects HEK proliferation, differentiation, and basal cell response(s) to sulfur mustard toxicity. The system will subsequently be used for testing the efficacy of prophylactic and therapeutic compounds.

MATERIALS AND METHODS

Epidermal Separation and Dissociation

Day-old human skin resections from the Cooperative Human Tissue Network (Ohio State University Research Foundation, Columbus, OH) were processed using aseptic techniques. Skin sections were trimmed of excess fat and connective tissue to a thickness of <2 mm, and were cut into pieces measuring approx 1 cm^2. Trimmed pieces were rinsed in Ham's F-12 containing gentamicin sulfate (50 µg/mL), then placed in 60-mm Petri dishes (6–8/dish), and incubated overnight at 6°C with dispase (Collaborative Biomedical Products, Bedford, MA). The proteolytic methods used were modified from those of S. Dan Dimitrijevich, Ph.D. (Department of Biochemistry and Molecular Biology, The University of North Texas Health Science Center at Fort Worth—personal communication) and from Haake and Lane *(15)*. Dispase activity was adjusted to 10 U/mL in mixed solutions of phosphate buffered saline (PBS; w/o Ca^{2+} and Mg^{2+}) and keratinocyte growth medium (KGM); Clonetics, San Diego, CA. Epidermal sheets were peeled from the dermis, then rinsed (1X), and triturated in trypsin-EDTA (0.05%–0.01%, Sigma Chemical Co., St. Louis, MO) for 15 min at room temperature. Dissociated cells (HEK) were suspended in DMEM containing 5% fetal bovine serum (FBS) and subjected to hemocytometer counts, then centrifuged for 10 min at 150*g*, and resuspended in fresh KGM. Primary cultures were prepared by inoculating 20,000–40,000 cells/cm² into 75-cm² tissue-culture flasks (Corning Glass Works, Corning, NY). The flasks were pretreated with FNC, a bovine fibronectin, collagen, and serum albumin substrate (Biological Research Faculty and Facility, Inc., Ijamsville, MD). When 65–85% confluent, primary cultures were either cryopreserved or subcultured.

Microscopy

Untreated, dispase-treated and epidermal skin sections (1 cm²) were immersed for 2 h at 5°C in Karnovsky's fixative consisting of 1.6% formaldehyde and 2.5% glutaraldehyde in 0.1 *M* sodium cacodylate. Fixed tissues were washed three times with cacodylate buffer (pH = 7.34), then postfixed in 1% osmium tetroxide for 15 min, dehydrated in graded ethanols, and embedded in epoxy resin. Semithin (1 μm) sections were cut and stained with Humphrey's stain (a mixture of methylene blue, azure II, and basic fuchsin) for light microscopy. Ultrathin (100-nm) sections were cut and counterstained with uranyl acetate and lead citrate, and then subjected to ultrastructural analysis by transmission electron microscopy (TEM) using a JEOL 1200 EX electron microscope.

Development of HEK Experimental Cultures

First-passage HEK were grown as (1) cocultures on feeder layers of 3T3 mouse fibroblasts pretreated with 4 μg/mL mitomycin-C (Sigma Chemical Co., St. Louis, MO), and as (2) pure cultures on FNC-coated glass cover slips. In coculture, HEK were maintained for 1 wk by methods modified from Rheinwald and Green *(16)* and from Mol *(17)*. The starter medium was a high calcium (1.43 m*M*) 3:1 mixture of DMEM: Ham's F-12 containing 5% FBS, 0.4 μg/mL hydrocortisone, 10 ng/mL epidermal growth factor (EGF), 10^{-10} *M* cholera toxin,

4 mM L-glutamine, and gentamicin sulfate (50 µg/mL). On day 7, the 3T3(s) were removed by vigorous aspiration, and the medium was replaced with low-calcium (0.15 mM) KGM. HEK in pure cultures were fed on KGM from day 1. Medium was renewed on alternate days in all cultures.

Bromodeoxyuridine (BrdU) Uptake and Distribution in Keratinocyte Cultures

HEK grown from cocultures were pulse-labeled with the thymidine analog BrdU at 24 and 48 h after removal of the 3T3 feeder layers. HEK were subsequently fixed at −20°C with 70% ethanol and stained with an anti-BrdU fluorescein tag using a BrdU-labeling kit (Boehringer Mannheim, Indianapolis, IN; cat. no. 1-296-736). Fluorescent images were produced and recorded on an ACAS-570 confocal microscope (Meridian Instruments, Okemos, MI) by scanning the control and BrdU-labeled HEK populations with a 488 laser line.

Indo-1AM Loading and Fluorescence from HD-Exposed Keratinocyte Cultures

Two to 3 d after removal of the 3T3 feeder layers, HEK were incubated with 1 µM Indo-1AM (Molecular Probes, Eugene, OR) for 1 h (at 35°C, 5% CO_2, 95% relative humidity) in PBS containing 1.02 mM Ca^{2+}. The HEK were then washed free of excess stain, exposed for 5 min to sulfur mustard (400 µM), and returned to either a low- (0.15 mM) or high- (1.02 mM) calcium buffer. Fluorescent images of control and HD-exposed populations were produced on an ACAS-570 confocal microscope by scanning with a 355 laser line.

RESULTS

Epidermal tissues were easily removed from human skin resections following an overnight incubation in dispase (Fig. 1). Histology of the skin before and after proteolytic treatment with dispase (Fig. 2) showed that overnight incubation produced microvesicles along the dermal/epidermal border, which facilitated sloughing and easy removal of the epidermis.

Details obtained by TEM showed that the microvesicles and separations produced by dispase occurred at the basement membrane along the line of the lamina densa (Fig. 3).

Epidermal tissues, when dissociated in trypsin/EDTA (0.05%/0.01%), produced average HEK yields that varied inversely with donor age (Fig. 4).

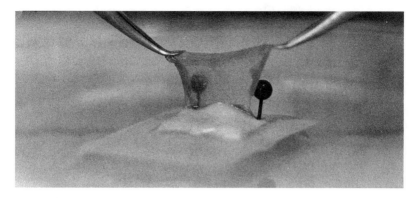

Fig. 1. Separation of the epidermis from whole skin. Overnight incubation of human skin at 6°C in 10 U/mL of dispase was used for proteolytic separation of dermal and epidermal tissues. Epidermal edges were easily lifted with a pair of fine forceps, and the entire tissue sheet was stripped clean of the underlying dermis.

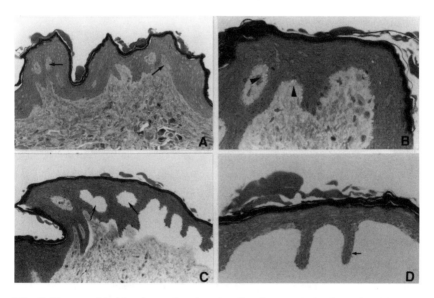

Fig. 2. Human skin histology showing details of proteolytic dermal/epidermal separations. Section of skin prior to dispase treatment (**A**) shows continuity of the dermal/epidermal border, including tangential and vertical cuts through the dermal papillae (arrows). Section taken 18 h after incubation with dispase (**B**) shows the formation of microvesicles along the dermal/epidermal border (arrowheads). Partial sloughing of the epidermis at 18 h after treatment with dispase (**C**) produced clean separations at the dermal/epidermal border with removal of dermal papillae from their insertions in the epidermis (arrows). When fully separated, the epidermis (**D**) constituent keratinocytes and rete peg architecture (arrow) remained intact (magnification A and C = 130×; B and D = 260×).

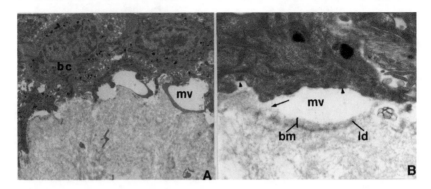

Fig. 3. Ultrastructural details of human skin (**A** and **B**) show microvesicles (mv) produced by incubation with dispase, and separation of basal cells (bc) from their basement membrane (bm) along the line of the lamina densa (ld). Basal cells are easily recognized by the presence of dense, cytoplasmic hemidesmosomes (arrow heads) and by their tonofilaments (arrow), which project into the basement membrane. (Magnification = 8000× and 40,000× for **A** and **B**, respectively).

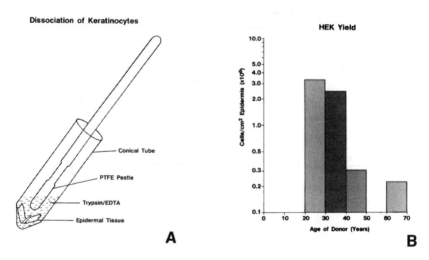

Fig. 4. Dissociation of HEK by triturating epidermal tissues in trypsin/EDTA (**A**). The histogram (**B**) shows that yields were as high as 3.5×10^6 HEK/cm^2 when tissues were obtained from young donors (20–40 yr old, $N = 8$). Yields from older donors were greatly reduced ($N = 5$).

Freshly dissociated and first-passage HEK produced compact colonies when grown in culture on either 3T3 feeder layers or FNC (Fig. 5). Colonies grown on FNC were compact with cells of similar size and shape. Colonies grown on feeder layers were complex and gave rise to

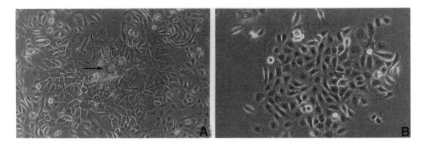

Fig. 5. HEK colonies grown from freshly dissociated human epidermal tissues. Colony formed on feeder layer of 3T3 mouse fibroblasts (**A**) showing core of stratified cells (arrow) and surroundings of spreading keratinocytes. When grown on FNC in KGM, a low-calcium (0.15 m*M*) medium, colonies did not produce a core of stratified cells (**B**).

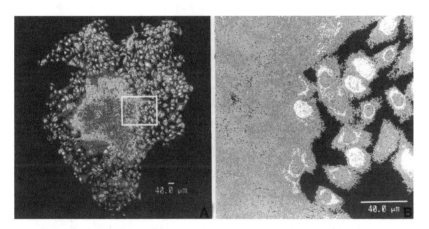

Fig. 6. HEK colony pulse labeled with BrdU and stained with fluorescein-tagged anti-BrdU. Two days after removal of 3T3 feeder layers, confocal images showed that proliferation was extensive, but was confined to cells at the perimeter of each colony (**A**). Nuclei of replicating cells were brightly fluorescent (**B**—enlargement).

a core of stratified cells with a surrounding layer of larger, flatter, peripheral keratinocytes. When the latter were pulse-labeled with BrdU and stained with fluorescein-tagged anti-BrdU, image analyses showed that only the peripheral cells incorporated BrdU (Fig. 6).

With colonies of cocultured HEK, there was also selective loading of Indo-1AM such that expression of Indo-1 fluorescence was restricted to the peripheral cells. Image analyses showed that HEK exposed to 400 µ*M*

HD in a low- (0.15-mM) calcium environment retained the features (size and shape) of control cells. Images also showed that acute exposure to high- (1.02 mM) calcium and to HD caused peripheral HEK to become larger, flatter, more angular, and crowded, and to increase their selective permeability for (leakage of) the Indo-1 probe (data not shown—*see 1*).

DISCUSSION

Despite the substantial yields of HEK obtained by proteolytic dissociation of the epidermis, only a small percent of the freshly isolated cells were high-efficiency colony formers in primary culture. However, these self-replicating stem cells gave rise to entire populations of HEK having a programmed capacity for growth and differentiation. Controlled expression of that potential is the basis for development of this model and for its use in testing our hypothesis that calcium involvement may affect sulfur mustard toxicity and the targeting of basal cells for vesicating lesions. When grown on FNC-coated tissue-culture plastics in a low-calcium (0.15-mM) medium, HEK stem cells showed no evidence of epidermal stratification or stacking of differentiated cells. By contrast, when HEK were initiated in 3T3 cocultures with a high-calcium medium (1.43 mM), a large majority of the colonies produced a central core of stratified cells. That core was maintained for at least several days after removal of the feeder layer and during proliferation of the colony's constituent cells in a low-calcium medium (KGM). We know that precursor basal cells stop cycling in vivo as they lift off the basement membrane and start climbing the calcium gradient of the epidermis *(8)*. Under normal physiological conditions, these transient cells are stimulated by epidermal calcium gradients to make autocrine and paracrine factors that trigger expression of specific cytokeratins, adhesion molecules, involucrin, and other markers of programmed differentiation. However, at some critical stage of differentiation, HEK lose their capacity to respond to calcium. Observations by Werrlein et al. *(1)* from images of peripheral cells in HEK colonies loaded with Indo-1AM indicate that cell size and shape can be altered dramatically by acute exposure to high calcium (1.02 mM), and that the permeability of proliferating cells increased when simultaneously exposed to high calcium and 400-μM sulfur mustard. Based on those observations and the proven existence of epidermal calcium gradients *(9,11)*, we have proposed that proliferating basal cells may be prime targets for sulfur mustard toxicity, because they are undifferentiated and programmed for response to small changes in their calcium environment. Using confocal microscopy, we have demonstrated that among HEK colonies developed in our coculture system, only the peripheral cells incorporate BrdU and proliferate when growing in a low-calcium medium. In that sense, they are like basal cells. Experiments are in progress using this model to test our hypothesis on calcium as a cofactor in mechanisms targeting basal cells for sulfur mustard toxicity.

ACKNOWLEDGMENT

The authors thank John Petrali for his professional courtesy, for the gracious use of his laboratory facilities, and for his expertise and assistance with the electron microscopy.

REFERENCES

1. Werrlein RJ, Madren-Whalley JS, Kirby SD, Mol M. Confocal microscopy and calcium images of keratinocytes exposed to sulfur mustard. In: Salem H, Katz SA, ed. Alternatives to Animal Toxicity, Taylor Francis, Washington, DC, 1998, pp. 409–416.
2. Hennings H, Michael D, Cheng C, Steinert P, Holbrook K, Yuspa S. Calcium regulation of growth and differentiation of mouse epidermal cells in culture. Cell 1980;19:245–254.
3. Hennings H, Holbrook KA. Calcium regulation of cell-cell contact and differentiation of epidermal cells in culture. Exp Cell Res 1983;143:127–142.
4. Hennings H, Kruszewski FH, Yuspa SH, Tucker RW. Intracellular calcium alterations in response to increased external calcium in normal and neoplastic keratinocytes. Carcinogenesis 1989;10:777–780.
5. Kruszewski FH, Hennings H, Yuspa SH, Tucker RW. Regulation of intracellular free calcium in normal murine keratinocytes. Am J Physiol 1991;261(Cell Physiol 30):C767–C773.
6. O'Keefe EJ, Payne RE. Modulation of the epidermal growth factor receptor of human keratinocytes by calcium ion. J Invest Dermatol 1983;81:231–235.
7. Stanley JR, Yuspa SH. Specific epidermal protein markers are modulated during calcium-induced terminal differentiation. J Cell Biol 1983;96:1809–1814.
8. Whitfield JF. Calcium as differentiator and killer-keratinocytes. In: Whitfield JF, ed. Calcium in Cell Cycles and Cancer. CRC, New York, 1995, pp. 123–151.
9. Menon GK, Grayson S, Elias PM. Ionic calcium reservoirs in mammalian epidermis: ultrastructural localization by ion-capture cytochemistry. J Invest Dermatol 1985;84:508–512.
10. Malmqvist KG, Forslind B, Roomans GM, Akelsson KR. Proton and electron microprobe analysis of human skin. Nucl Instr Meth Res 1984;B3:611–617.
11. Forslind Bo. Particle probe analysis in the study of skin physiology. In: Scanning Electron Microsc 3:1007–1014. Symposium on Cell Structure and Cell Biology in honor of Björn Afzelius, Dec. 19–20, Stockholm, Sweden, 1986.
12. Menon GK, Elias PM, Feingold KR. Integrity of the permeability barrier is crucial for maintenance of the epidermal calcium gradient. Br J Dermatol 1994;130:139–147.
13. Grundin TG, Roomans GM, Forslind Bo, Lindberg M, Werner Y. X-ray microanalysis of psoriatic skin. J Invest Dermatol 1985;85:378-380.

14. Menon GK, Elias PM. Ultrastructural localization of calcium in psoriatic and normal human epidermis. Arch Dermatol 1991;127:57–63.
15. Haake AR, Lane AT. Retention of differentiated characteristics in human fetal keratinocytes *in vitro*. In Vitro, Cell Dev Biol 1989;25:592–600.
16. Rheinwald JG, Green H. Serial cultivation of strains of human epidermal keratinocytes: the formation of keratinizing colonies from single cells. Cell 1975; 6:331–344.
17. Mol MAE. Changes in intracellular free calcium levels of cultured human epidermal keratinocytes exposed to sulfur mustard, vol. 1. In: Proceedings of the 1993 Medical Defense Bioscience Review. United States Army Medical Research Institute of Chemical Defense, Aberdeen Proving Ground, MD. AD-275 667, 1993, pp. 277–283.

15 Phosgene-Induced Calcium Changes in Pulmonary Artery Endothelial Cells

Robert J. Werrlein, PhD, Stephen D. Kirby, BS and Janna S. Madren-Whalley

CONTENTS

INTRODUCTION

Phosgene ($COCl_2$) is a severe respiratory irritant. Inhalation of the gas disrupts fluid balance in the lung, causes acute pulmonary edema, and can potentiate immunosuppression and opportunistic infections even at low doses. Although phosgene has been used as a weapon of war, the primary medical concern regarding treatment of injuries caused by phosgene is largely about issues of occupational health. According to NIOSH [1], more than 10,000 workers are employed annually to produce and transport 1 million tons of phosgene in essential support of our nation's chemical industries. We know from EPA concerns that in the production process, 80,000 pounds are released each year into the ambient air [2]. Clinical reports on occupational health indicate that respiratory injuries sustained from work with welding equipment, paint removers, and various chlorinated solvents [3,4] have been the result of phosgene inhalation and that such incidents occur more frequently than commonly expected. Despite the hazards posed by accidental or inten-

From: *Toxicity Assessment Alternatives: Methods, Issues, Opportunities*
Edited by: H. Salem and S. A. Katz © Humana Press Inc., Totowa, NJ

tional release of phosgene, there is still very little known about the pathophysiology of phosgene toxicity, and there is no certain postexposure treatment for inhalation victims. Previously we reported *(5)* that phosgene effects changes in F-actin concentration and organization in cells grown from sheep and rat lungs. Those cytoskeletal effects occurred within 20 min of exposure, were dose-dependent, and showed cell-specific sensitivity. In the following study, we demonstrate that calcium changes occur very early during in vitro exposures to phosgene and probably prior to changes in F-actin.

MATERIALS AND METHODS

Cell Cultures

Sheep pulmonary arterial endothelial cells (PAECs) in low passage (6–10) were seeded at 10,000–20,000 cells/cm^2 in glass-bottomed microwells precoated with 30 μg/cm^2 type I collagen (Vitrogen 100, Collagen Corp., Palo Alto, CA). Cells were sustained on Ham's F-12 medium containing 15% FBS, 50 μg/mL endothelial cell growth factor, 2 mM L-glutamine (Sigma Chemical Company, St. Louis, MO) plus 50 μg/mL gentamicin sulfate (Whittaker M.A. Bioproducts, Walkersville, MD) and 5% Omni™, a serum supplement (Advanced Biotechnologies Inc., Columbia, MD). Cultures were grown at 35°C in a humidified atmosphere of 5% CO$_2$ and air, and were subjected to daily medium renewal. Populations were subconfluent and 2- to 4-d old at time of experiment.

Loading Cells with INDO-1AM

Cultures were washed 2× with Ham's F-12 (without phenol red and serum), then incubated at 35°C for 1 h with 1 μM Indo 1-AM (Molecular Probes, Eugene, OR) in 2 mL of PBS containing Ca^{2+} and Mg^{2+} salts. The supernatant and unincorporated dye were discarded, and the cells were washed 2× with prewarmed Ham's F-12 (as above).

Phosgene Exposures

Experimental cultures, preloaded with Indo-1AM, were placed in a specially constructed environmental chamber designed for real-time studies of cellular response to phosgene. Cells in the microwell were covered with 12 μL of F-12 medium (without serum and phenol red), and then sealed in the chamber. That amount of medium kept the cells wet and maintained their osmolarity and pH. During exposure, the environmental chamber was placed on the stage of an Meridian ACAS-570 confocal laser microscope (Genomic Solutions Inc., Lansing, MI). Phosgene (40 μL = 228 ppm) was injected into the chamber and mixed by microfan at the start of each 20-min exposure. Hydrolysis and decreased phosgene concentration were determined over time by gas chromatography using a chromsil 310 column (Supelco, Inc., Bellefonte, PA) and HP 5880A gas chromatograph (Hewlett Packard, Palo Alto, CA) to analyze chamber gas samples. Sham-control populations were subjected to 40 μL of air, and all exposures were conducted in a humidified atmosphere of 5% CO_2 and air.

Image and Calcium Analysis

X-Z image scans (cross-sections of cells) were run at 15-s intervals throughout the course of each 20-min exposure producing 75 fluorescent image pairs/experiment. Excitation (355-nm laser line) and emission wavelengths were separated by dichroic beam splitting mirrors. The 485-nm, Ca^{2+}-free Indo-1 emissions were recorded by detector #1, and the 405-nm, Ca^{2+}-bound Indo-1 emissions were recorded by detector #2. Time plots were generated to show response patterns associated with phosgene-induced changes in Ca^{2+}-free and Ca^{2+}-bound Indo-1 emissions. Intracellular free calcium concentrations and calcium kinetics were determined by analysis of the successive detector #2:detector #1 image ratios, and by use of calibration curves constructed at the end of each experiment with calcium standards and the same parameters (PMT sensitivity settings, and so forth) that were used for the experiment. Field scans were run prior to and following exposure to determine whether phosgene induced detectable calcium changes in entire fields of cells.

RESULTS

X-Z image scans of sham-control populations, i.e., cells subjected to room air under controlled environmental conditions, showed no visible shift of fluorescence (image) intensity between detector #1 and detector #2. Graphic presentation of the corresponding calcium results (time plots and ratio analyses), as seen in Fig. 1, indicated that repeated laser scans (n =75) produced some photobleaching, but without substantially altering the emissions from detectors #1 and #2. Quantitation by ratio analysis of the image sequences (detector #2:detector #1) indicated that intracellular free calcium for PAECs under the experimental conditions was approx 50–60 nM.

In untreated controls and pre-exposed populations, the brightest intracellular calcium images were obtained from 485 nm (Ca^{2+}-free Indo-1) emissions recorded by detector #1. In postexposure comparison

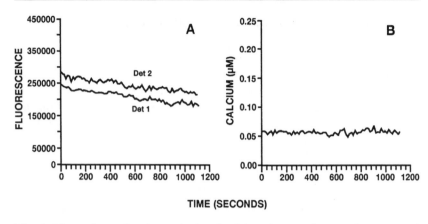

TIME (SECONDS)

Fig. 1. Time plot and ratio analysis of calcium images from a sham-control population. X-Z image scans were recorded at 15-s intervals during a 20-min control experiment in which PAECs were challenged with 40 μL of air under controlled environmental conditions. Sham-exposures produced no visible shift of fluorescence intensity from detector #1 to detector #2, or vice versa. (A) A time plot of fluorescent emissions from the successive X-Z scans ($n = 75$ image pairs) indicates some photobleaching, but no real change in detector #1 (485 nm, Ca^{2+}-free Indo-1) or detector #2 (405 nm, Ca^{2+}-bound Indo-1) emissions. (B) Ratio analysis of the same (detector #2:detector #1) images shows a basal, free-calcium concentration of 50–60 nM throughout the experiment.

of the same cell fields, real-time responses to phosgene showed that fluorescence intensity of calcium images shifted visibly from detector #1 to detector #2, and usually but not always recovered. The shift in fluorescence intensity has been recorded for entire fields of PAECs, which indicates that many cells in these endothelial populations respond to phosgene exposure by elevating and sometimes maintaining higher levels of intracellular free calcium. However, the usual response was short-lived, and there was detectable variation among individual cells.

X-Z image scans ($n = 75$), recorded during exposure of PAECs to sublethal doses of phosgene, showed that with some cells phosgene caused an early decrease in 485-nm emissions from Ca^{2+}-free Indo-1 (detector #1) and a reciprocal increase in 405-nm emissions from Ca^{2+}-bound Indo-1 (detector #2). In Fig. 2, the visible increase of intra-cellular free calcium peaked at T = 60 s of exposure and partial recovery occurred within 240 s.

Under exposure of PAECs to a single burst of phosgene (228 ppm), we determined that in culture, isolated cells were capable of multiple calcium responses. In the examples shown (Figs. 3 and 4), four distinct calcium peaks were recorded from a single cell over a 20-min (1200 s)

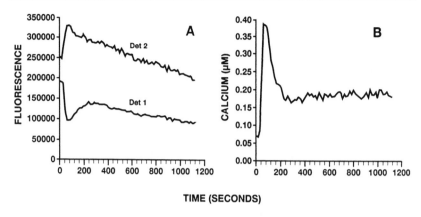

TIME (SECONDS)

Fig. 2. Time plot and ratio analysis of calcium images from a population exposed to phosgene. (A) A time plot of the fluorescence recorded by detector #1 and detector #2 during sublethal exposure to phosgene indicates that in the PAEC under investigation the calcium response was initiated within 20 s of injecting phosgene (228 ppm) into the exposure chamber. In A, the graphics show a rapid rise of fluorescence in detector #2, a concomitant decrease of fluorescence in detector #1 and a partial recovery. The reciprocal peaks were nearly equal in amplitude and duration. Peak rise-time was 40 s, peak duration 20 s, and recovery 160 s. (B) Ratio analysis of (detector #2:detector #1) images confirmed that the calcium response to phosgene was a substantial, early event. During the initial 60 s of exposure (196 ppm/min), intracellular free calcium increased 5.5-fold from 70–386 nM. Partial recovery ended with an elevated basal concentration of 190 nM free calcium, which was sustained throughout the experiment.

exposure period. The initial calcium response at T = 60 s and the next at T = 240 s produced reciprocal deflections by detector #1 and detector #2 that were nearly equal in amplitude and duration. Peak amplitude of the third calcium response was reduced in size but its rise time (40 s) and duration (100 s) were similar. The last response of the series was incomplete.

In some PAEC populations, calcium response to phosgene was protracted, and the changes in 485 nm (detector #1) and 405 nm (detector #2) emissions were not obviously reciprocal. As shown in Fig. 5A, such responses were characterized by Ca^{2+}-bound Indo-1 (405 nm) emissions that remained quite stable at the expense of rapidly degrading Ca^{2+}-free Indo-1 (485-nm) emissions.

Comparison of real-time responses to phosgene showed that the fluorescence intensity of calcium images shifted visibly from Ca^{2+}-free to Ca^{2+}-bound Indo-1 (i.e., from detector #1 to detector #2) and usually, but not always, recovered. This shift in fluorescence intensity has been

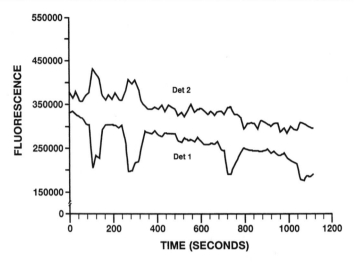

Fig. 3. Multiple calcium responses during exposure to phosgene. Time plot of a calcium response by a PAEC to a single burst of phosgene (228 ppm) shows that the initial response occurred at T = 60 s of exposure (196 ppm/min), peaked at 105 s after a substantial increase in 405 nm (Ca^{2+}-bound Indo-1; detector #2) emissions and a reciprocal decrease in 485 nm (Ca^{2+}-free Indo-1; detector #1) emissions. Nearly full recovery was achieved in the ensuing 55 s. The second response at T = 240 s (80 s later) began in an atmosphere containing ~84 ppm phosgene, and produced reciprocal detector responses (fluorescent peaks) that were nearly equal in amplitude and duration to the initial calcium response. The third response at T = 690 s (after a delay of 6 min) began in an atmosphere containing ~25 ppm phosgene. Peak amplitude of the response was reduced, but rise time (40 s) and duration of calcium flux (100 s) were similar to previous responses. The fourth response was interrupted by completion of the timed experiment.

recorded for entire fields of PAECs, which indicates that many cells in these endothelial populations respond to phosgene exposure by elevating and sometimes maintaining higher levels of intracellular free calcium. Therefore, although typical responses were short-lived, there was detectable variation among individual cells.

DISCUSSION

Real-time ratio analysis of Ca^{2+}-bound and Ca^{2+}-free Indo-1 emissions showed that exposure to sublethal doses of phosgene produced early, substantial increases of intracellular free calcium. Responses varied among individual PAECs indicating that in subconfluent (proliferating) populations, cell-cycle kinetics might affect mechanisms controlling calcium mobilization. In pre-exposed and sham-control

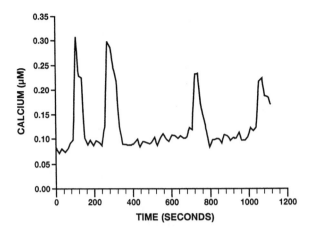

Fig. 4. Calcium concentrations during multiple responses to phosgene. Ratio analysis of the data presented in Fig. 3 shows that prior to the initial response, intracellular free calcium had equilibrated at a concentration of 75 n*M*. During the initial T = 60 s response to phosgene (196 ppm/min), there was a fourfold calcium increase to 300 n*M* and a recovery to 93 n*M*. The second peak response (with phosgene hydrolyzed to 84 ppm) produced a 3.1-fold increase from 93 to 289 n*M* and a recovery to 89 n*M*. Through the ensuing 6 min, there was a gradual rise of intracellular free calcium to 100 n*M*. In response #3, intracellular free calcium peaked at 225 n*M* and recovered to 89 n*M*.

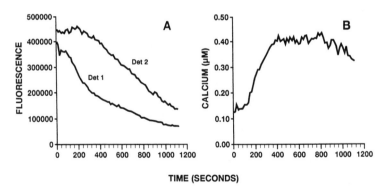

Fig. 5. Protracted calcium response to phosgene. **(A)** Real-time analysis (time plot) of a PAEC response to phosgene shows that the Ca^{2+}-bound Indo-1 (detector #2) fluorescence remained fairly stable for 240 s before there was a decline in the corresponding 405-nm emissions. There were no reciprocal peak emissions; however, the initial stability of detector #2 fluorescence was coincident with a precipitous decrease in the 485-nm, detector #1 emissions. **(B)** Ratio analysis indicates that intracellular free calcium began to increase at T= 60 s and rose from 125 to 410 n*M* during the next 6 min of exposure. However, the apparent 3.28-fold increase of intracellular free calcium is a product of ratio analyses based on the disproportionate and unaccountable early decreases in Ca^{2+}-free Indo-1 emissions.

populations, bathed in 1.02 mM extracellular calcium, basal calcium levels were relatively low (60–125 nM). Phosgene induced calcium peak responses of 300 to 410 nM and produced transient free calcium increases of up to 5.5-fold. Most transients peaked within 15–30 s, i.e., the time required for 1–2 successive image scans. It is not certain whether phosgene triggered a release of internal Ca^{2+} stores or whether it caused external Ca^{2+} to be imported through channels in the plasma membrane. Given the steep ~10,000-fold difference in calcium concentration between the extracellular and cytosolic spaces, any perturbation of the membrane by phosgene might produce substantial calcium penetration and a significant, although transient increase of intracellular free calcium. However, the image patterns and rate of response indicate that phosgene may have triggered some second messenger mechanism linked to mobilization of calcium stores and not to a breach in integrity of plasma membrane permeability. In fact, the uniform and consistently central localization of fluorescence in X-Z image scans, both at rest and throughout the peaking of calcium transients (Figs. 2, 3, and 4), favors a mechanism based on mobilization of internal stores. We suggest that if the plasma membrane that has evolved as a barrier to protect cytosolic targets from high calcium concentrations had been breached, X-Z scans should have captured bright fluorescent images propagating along the membrane margins. They did not. Although the mechanisms remain uncertain, intracellular free calcium could be accurately assessed from peak responses that were reciprocal and without unusual depletion of the Indo-1 probe. However, the 3.28-fold increase in intracellular free calcium in Fig. 5 remains in question, because the ratio analyses were based on disproportionate and unaccountably large decreases in 485 nm, Ca^{2+}-free Indo-1 (detector #1) emissions. We have speculated that under physiological conditions that give rise to protracted and nonreciprocal detector responses, phosgene might induce a low-affinity calcium turnover (calcium activity) with stoichiometric discharge of Ca^{2+}-bound Indo-1 from the PAECs and concomitant import of free calcium. Through dynamic exchange, an influx of free calcium might complex with and deplete the Ca^{2+}-free Indo-1 stores (485-nm emissions), thus maintaining the 405 nm fluorescent output of Ca^{2+}-bound Indo-1 without actually increasing intracellular free calcium concentrations.

CONCLUSIONS

- Under controlled environmental conditions, exposure to phosgene (196 ppm/min) produced early and substantial increases of intracellular free calcium among sheep pulmonary artery endothelial cells in culture.

- Real-time ratio analysis of $(Ca^{2+}$-bound) : $(Ca^{2+}$-free) Indo-1 emissions showed that phosgene induced intracellular free calcium increases of up to 5.5-fold (70–386 nM) within 40–60 s of exposure.
- Calcium response to phosgene varied among cells in proliferating PAEC populations.
- Responses to phosgene can involve single or multiple calcium events with full or partial recovery and may involve different regulatory mechanisms.

REFERENCES

1. National Institute for Occupational Safety and Health (NIOSH). Occupational exposure to phosgene. US Department of Health, Education and Welfare, US Government Printing Office, Washington DC, Publication no. 76-137 (NIOSH), 1976, pp. 1–129.
2. National Toxic Release Inventory. US Congress Subcommittee on Health and the Environment. Henry A. Waxman (Chairman), 1989.
3. Sjögren B, Plato N, Alexandersson R, Eklund A, Falkenberg C. Pulmonary reactions caused by welding-induced decomposed trichlorethylene. Chest 1991;99: 237,238.
4. Snyder RW, Mishel HS, Christensen, GC. Pulmonary toxicity following exposure to methylene chloride and its combustion product, phosgene. Chest 1992;101: 860,861.
5. Werrlein RJ, Madren-Whalley JS, Kirby SD. Phosgene effects on F-actin organization and concentration in cells cultured from sheep and rat lung. Cell Biol Toxicol 1994;10:45–58.

16 Enhanced Proteolytic Activity and Fc Receptor Expression in Human Epithelial Cells Following Exposure to Sulfur Mustard

Fred M. Cowan, BSc,
Clarence A. Broomfield, PhD,
and William J. Smith, PhD

CONTENTS

INTRODUCTION
MATERIALS AND METHODS
RESULTS
DISCUSSION
REFERENCES

INTRODUCTION

Nearly a century of investigation of sulfur mustard (HD) (2,2'-dichloro-diethyl sulfide) has yielded only theoretical explanations of the toxicological mechanisms of this compound *(1,2)*. Presently, no biochemical marker can predict the histopathological changes associated with HD toxicity and no antidote exists *(1–3)*. Much of the information pertaining to HD cutaneous pathology is derived from clinical observations of exposed subjects *(2,4)*. The basic histopathology of HD-induced cutaneous lesions includes the formation of vesicles at the dermal–epidermal junction *(1,2)*. The resemblance of the cutaneous injury produced by HD to that caused by proteolysis suggests that HD-increased proteolytic activity might contribute to HD toxicity *(1,2)*. Papirmeister and

From: *Toxicity Assessment Alternatives: Methods, Issues, Opportunities*
Edited by: H. Salem and S. A. Katz © Humana Press Inc., Totowa, NJ

coworkers *(1)* have proposed that HD alkylates DNA, causing DNA strand breakage and leading to subsequent biochemical and metabolic alterations that culminate in enhancement of proteolytic activity in epithelial cells. Furthermore, proteolytic enzymes associated with the inflammatory response may exacerbate the cutaneous lesion and contribute to blister formation *(2,3)*.

Enhanced proteolysis of chromogenic peptide substrates has been reported following in vitro exposure of rabbit skin cul¿9res *(5)*, human peripheral blood lymphocytes (PBL) *(6)*, human skin equivalent, Testskin®, and epidermal keratinocytes to HD *(7)*. In vivo exposure of hairless guinea pig skin to HD causes increased proteolytic activity *(8)* that is consistent with the time-course of the appearance of HD pathology *(3,9)*. Niacinamide, an inhibitor of poly(ADP-ribose) polymerase, prevents HD-induced NAD⁺ depletion and may restore some normal metabolic activities in HD-exposed cells *(10)*. Niacinamide also decreases both cytotoxicity *(10)* and proteolysis *(11)* in PBL cell cultures exposed to HD, and can reduce HD-induced microvesicle formation in hairless guinea pigs *(12)*.

The enzyme myeloperoxidase *(13)* and the proteolytic enzyme elastase *(3)* are markers for leukocyte infiltration, and increases in these and other enzymes have been detected in soluble extracts from HD-exposed hairless guinea pig skin *(11)*. The cytotoxic drug hydroxyurea inhibits DNA synthesis in both immune and skin cells, and can decrease white blood cell counts *(14,15)*. Phenidone antagonizes arachidonic acid metabolites and the cutaneous neutrophil infiltration associated with inflammation *(16)*. HD-increased proteolysis measured in extracts of hairless guinea pig skin biopsies was practically eliminated by systemic treatment with hydroxyurea and was greatly diminished by topical application of the anti-inflammatory drug phenidone *(17;* Bongiovani et al., personal communication). HD-increased proteolysis in cell cultures *(6,7)* and inflammatory enzymes in HD-exposed hairless guinea pig skin *(8,13)* indicate that metabolic disruption of skin cells and/or inflammation could contribute to HD pathology *(1–3)*. Therefore, the study of HD-increased proteolysis and expression of immune molecules, such as receptors for the Fc region of antibody (FcR), in human keratinocyte cell cultures may provide biomarkers that might be used to elucidate both the toxicological action of and antidotes for HD.

MATERIALS AND METHODS

Peptide Substrates and Reagents

The Chromozym® substrate TRY (enzyme specificity, trypsin-like) was purchased from Boehringer Mannheim Biochemicals, Indianapolis, IN. HD with a purity of >98% was obtained from the US Army Edgewood Research, Development and Engineering Center, Aberdeen Proving Ground, MD. Human epidermal keratinocyte (HEK)and keratinocyte growth media (KGM) were purchased from Clonetics, San Diego, CA.

Keratinocytes

HEK were grown to 100% confluence using KGM in 24-well tissue-culture plates for assay of proteolysis and 96-well plates for immune fluorescence.

Sulfur Mustard Exposure

HEK in 24-well tissue-culture plates at 100% confluence were exposed to 1 mL of 50–1000 μM HD/well. The plates were maintained at room temperature in a fume hood for 1 h to allow venting of volatile agent and then transferred to a CO_2 incubator at 37°C. At 2 h post-HD exposure, KGM media were reduced to 250 μL and returned to incubator for a total incubation time of 4–24 h.

Chromogenic Peptide Substrate Protease Assay

Chromogenic peptide substrates, when cleaved by protease, release p-nitroaniline (pNA), producing a change in absorbance measured spectrophotometrically at 405 nm (18). The use of these small proteolysis sensitive peptides was adapted for protease assay by microplate reader (Molecular Devices, CA) as previously described (6).

To HEK attached to 24-well plates with 100 μL of their supernants remaining was added 100 μL substrate (2.5 mM) for an assay concentration of 1.25 mM. The plates were then placed in a CO_2 incubator at 37°C for 1 h. Assay supernates (100 μL) were transferred to 96-well plates for reading absorbance. To eliminate background, absorbance readings were made on a microplate reader at 405 nM using media/substrate controls as blank values.

Immune Fluorescence of CD32

Anti-CD32-FITC antibody, and isotype controls were obtained from PharmMingen, San Diego, CA. Immune fluorescence assay was performed as previously described (19) and read on a Zeiss fluorescence microscope.

Data Analysis

All data points were assayed in duplicate. Data are presented from single experiments that are representative of other similar experiments,

Table 1
HD-Increased Proteolysis in HEK

Dose HD	Absorbance
Control	0.175 ± 0.009
50 µm	0.168 ± 0.014
100 µm	0.239 ± 0.010
200 µm	0.465 ± 0.027
500 µm	0.151 ± 0.029^{a}

[a]Value corrected from percent control; separate experiment.

Table 2
CD32 in HD-Exposed HEK

Hours post-HD	Dose HD, FITC, PE		
	50	100	200
8	$\pm^{a}$	$\pm$	$\pm$
24	+	++	+++

[a]Grading of staining: $\pm$, occasional; +, weak; ++, moderate; +++, intense as assayed by fluorescence microscopy.

and numerical data are expressed as mean of absorbance. Individual group significance was determined by Student's t-test, and absorbance data are presented with standard errors.

RESULTS

Exposure of HEK to 100 or 200 µM HD and assay with the TRY substrate showed a concentration-dependent increase in proteolysis above the baseline activity of unexposed controls (Table 1). In separate experiments, 500 µM HD did not increase proteolysis (Table 1), and a 1000-µm concentration of HD inhibited increased proteolysis below the baseline activity of unexposed controls (data not shown). HD-increased proteolysis in HEK was generally cell-associated, but was also often detected in culture supernants.

HD, in addition to increasing proteolysis, also caused time- and dose-dependent morphological changes. These changes included loss of "cobblestone" appearance of cultures, with diminished cell–cell contact and rounding of cells. The morphological changes were also associated with increased CD32 expression (Table 2).

DISCUSSION

Exposure of keratinocyte cell cultures to HD increases proteolysis in a concentration-dependent manner. HD-increased proteolytic activity is also time-dependent with increased proteolysis detected as early as 4 h after HD exposure and with maximum activity observed by 24 h *(7)*. This time frame correlates well with the ultrastructural demonstration of protease-like cleavage of adherent fibrils at the epidermal–dermal junction following HD exposure *(1,2)*.

Proteolysis or protease receptor interactions may contribute to the metabolic disruption and/or inflammation associated with HD exposure, and the skin immune response may involve direct participation of resident epithelial cells *(3)*. Proteases can act as ligand binding-specific receptors to alter metabolic functions and inflammation, and enhance expression of immune receptors *(20–22)*. For example, thrombin can act as an immune mediator, and can stimulate vascular endothelial cells to synthesize and transport platelet-activating factor to plasma membranes, resulting in maximum neutrophil adhesion *(21,22)*. Keratinocytes produce, and have receptors for a myriad of immune molecules to include cytokines and complement components, and HEK are known to express the FcR *(19,23,24)*. FcR bind to the Fc region of antibody, are found on all types of immune cells, and mediate many effector and regulatory functions *(25,26)*. Assay by microscope with anti-FcR fluorescent antibodies demonstrated that exposure of HEK to HD increased CD32 in a time- and concentration-dependent manner that was consistent with the appearance of HD-increased proteolysis and HD toxicity.

The CD32 FcR is known to be involved in cutaneous immune complex-mediated mast cell degranulation and complement activation that results in an immediate-type hypersensitivity "Arthus reaction" *(27,28)*. Cutaneous exposure to HD causes mast cell degranulation in the skin of hairless guinea pigs *(29)*. It is possible that HD-enhanced CD32 could cause an Arthus-like reaction wherein soluble inflammatory mediators of mast cell and complement activation could damage the epidermal junction and recruit further infiltration of inflammatory cells. This might be complicated by HD-increased protease binding to its receptor enhancing the expression of FcR or cleaving antibody to form Fc fragments that can activate FcR immunity *(30)*.

The potential for proteases to affect cell biochemistry and inflammatory responses may be relevant to both HD toxicity and the actions of drugs on HD pathology. For example, the anti-inflammatory drugs phenidone and dexamethasone suppress both inflammation and protease activity *(3,8,31,32)*, and vitamin D_3 (calciferol) can inhibit both proteolysis and FcR expression in HEK *(8,33,34)*. If HD-increased proteolysis and inflammatory response contribute to HD toxicity *(1–3)*, then HD-increased proteolytic activity and enhanced FcR expression in HEK cultures may prove useful for elucidating the mechanism(s) of HD-induced vesication. Ultimately, testing of compounds that reduce HD-increased proteolytic activity and/or FcR expression might further define the mechanisms of HD-induced cutaneous pathology and identify medical countermeasures for HD toxicity.

REFERENCES

1. Papirmeister B, Gross CL, Meier HL, Petrali JP, Johnson JB. Molecular basis for mustard-induced vesication. Fundam Appl Toxicol 1985;5:S134–S149.
2. Papirmeister B, Feister AJ, Robinson SI, Ford RD. In: Medical Defense Against Mustard Gas: Toxic Mechanisms and Pharmacological Implications. CRC, Boston, 1991, pp. 1–359.
3. Cowan FM, Broomfield CA. Putative roles of inflammation in the dermatopathology of sulfur mustard. Cell Biol Toxicol 1993;9:201–213.
4. Pechura CM, Rall DP, eds. Veterans at Risk: The Health Effects of Mustard Gas and Lewisite. National Academy Press, Washington DC, 1993.
5. Higuchi K, Kajiki A, Nakamura M, Harada S, Pula PJ, Scott AL, et al. Protease released in organ culture by acute inflammatory lesions produced in vivo in rabbit skin by sulfur mustard: hydrolysis of synthetic peptide substrates for trypsin-like and chymotrypsin-like enzymes. Inflammation 1988;12:311–334.
6. Cowan FM, Broomfield CA, Smith, WJ. Effect of sulfur mustard on protease activity in human peripheral blood lymphocytes. Cell Biol Toxicol 1991;7:239–248.
7. Smith WJ, Cowan FM, Broomfield CA. Increased proteolytic activity in human epithelial cells following exposure to sulfur mustard. FASEB J 1991;5:A828.
8. Cowan FM, Bongiovanni R, Broomfield CA, Yourick JJ, Smith WJ. Sulfur mustard increases elastase-like activities in homogenates of hairless guinea pig skin. J Toxicol-Cutaneous Ocular Toxicol 1994;13:221–229.
9. Cowan FM, Yourick JJ, Hurst CG, Broomfield CA, Smith WJ. Sulfur mustard-increased proteolysis following *in vitro* and *in vivo* exposures. Cell Biol Toxicol 1993;9:253–261.
10. Meier HL, Gross CL, Papirmeister B. 2,2'-Dichlorodiethyl sulfide (sulfur mustard) decreases NAD+ in human leukocytes. Toxicol Lett 1987;39:109–122.
11. Cowan FM, Broomfield CA, Smith WJ. Inhibition of sulfur mustard-increased protease activity by niacinamide, *N*-acetyl-L-cysteine or dexamethasone. Cell Biol Toxicol 1992;8:9–133.
12. Yourick JJ, Clark CR, Mitcheltree LW. Niacinamide pretreatment reduces microvesicle formation in hairless guinea pigs cutaneously exposed to sulfur mustard. Fundam Appl Toxicol 1991;17:622–630.
13. Bongiovanni R, Millard CB, Schulz SM, Romano JM. Estimation of neutrophil infiltration into hairless guinea pig skin treated with 2,2'-dichlorodiethyl sulfide. Proceedings of the 1993 Medical Defense Bioscience Review. USAMRICD, Aberdeen Proving Ground, Maryland, vol. 1, May 10–13, ADA275667, 1993, pp. 389–395.
14. Goodman LS, GilmanA, Gilman AG. The Pharmacological Basis of Therapeutics, 8th ed. Pergamon, New York, 1990, pp. 1251–1252.

15. Smith HC, Boutwell RK, Potter VR. Effects of hydroxyurea on DNA and RNA synthesis in mouse skin, liver, and thymus and on skin tumorigenesis initiated by α_{15}-propiolactone. Can Res 1968;28:2217–2227.

16. Harris RR, Mackin WM, Batt DG, Rakich SM, Collins RJ, Bruin EM, et al. Cellular and biochemical characterization of the anti-inflammatory effects of DuP654 in the arachidonic acid murine skin inflammation model. Skin Pharmacol 1990;3:29–40.

17. Cowan FM, Bongiovanni R, Broomfield CA, Schulz SM, Smith WJ. Phenidone and hydroxyurea reduce sulfur mustard-increased proteolysis in hairless guinea pig skin. J Toxicol-Cutaneous Ocular Toxicol 1994;14:265–272.

18. Friberger P. Chromogenic peptide substrates. Scand J Clin Lab Invest 1982;42(Suppl 162):1–98.

19. Tigalonowa M, Bjerke JR, Livden JK, Matre R. The distribution of FcRI, FcRII, and FcRIII on Langerhans' cells and keratinocytes in normal skin. Acta Derm Venereol (Stockh) 1990;70:385–390.

20. Chan IJ, Tharp MD. Rat mast cell protease I alters cell metabolism. J Invest Dermatol 1994;103:84–87.

21. Cirino G, Cicala C, Bucci MR, Sorrentino L, Maraganore JM, Stone SR. Thrombin functions as an inflammatory mediator through activation of its receptor. J Exp Med 1996;183:821–827.

22. Katayama H, Hase T, Yaoita H. Detachment of cultured normal human keratinocytes by contact with TNF-stimulated neutrophils in the presence of platelet-activating factor. J Invest Dermatol 1994;103:187–190.

23. Hunyadi J, Simon M Jr, Dobozy A. Immune-associated surface markers of human keratinocytes. Immunol Lett 1992;31:209–216.

24. Nunes IP, Johannesen AC, Matre R, Kristoffersen T. Epithelial expression of HLA class II antigens abd Fc receptors in patients with adult periodontitis. J Clin Periodontol 1994;21:256–232.

25. Ravetch JV. Fc receptors: rubor redux. Cell 1994;78:553–560.

26. Cowan FM, Madsen JM. The role of immunoglobulin binding factors in the pathogenesis and therapy of AIDS. Med Hypothesis 1994;43:172–176.

27. Sylvestre DL, Ravetch JV. Fc receptors initiate the arthus reaction: redefining the inflammatory cascade. Science 1994;265:1095–1098.

28. Frick OL. Immediate Hypersensitivity. In: Stites DP, Stobo JD, Wells JV, eds. Basic and Clinical Immunology, 6th ed. Appleton & Lange, CA, 1987, pp. 197–227.

29. Graham JS, Bryant MA, Braue EH. Effect of sulfur mustard on mast cells in hairless guinea pig skin. J Toxicol-Cutaneous Ocular Toxicol 1994;13:47–54.

30. Berman MA, Weigle WO. Lymphocyte stimulation with Fc fragments. J Immunol 1979;122:89–73.

31. Wilhelms OH, Linssen MJ, Lipponer L, Seilnaacht W. Nimesulide, indomethacin, BW755 C, phenidon, mepacrin and nedocromil inhibits the activation of human and rat leukocytes. Int J Tissue Reac 1990;XII:101–106.

32. Saunders PR, Marshall JS. Dexamethasone induces a down regulation of rat mast cell protease II content in rat basophilic leukaemia cells. Agents Actions 1992; 36:3–10.

33. Koli K, Keski-oja J. Vitamin D_3 and calcipotriol decrease extracellular plasminogen activator activity in cultured keratinocytes. J Invest Dermatol 1993;101:706–712.

34. Boltz-Nitulescu G, Willheim M, Spitter A, Leutmezer F, Tempfer C, Winkler S. Modulation of IgA, IgE, and IgG Fc receptor expression on human mononuclear phagocytes by 1a, 25-dihydroxyvitamin D^3. J Leukocyte Biol 1995;58:256–262.

17

Altered Expression of Intracellular and Surface Antigens by Cultured Human Epidermal Keratinocytes Exposed to Sulfur Mustard

William J. Smith, PhD

CONTENTS

INTRODUCTION
METHODS
RESULTS
DISCUSSION
REFERENCES

INTRODUCTION

Full understanding of the mechanisms of sulfur mustard (HD) toxicity has not yet been attained. Part of the problem rests with the high degree of reactivity of this alkylating agent and its multiple cellular targets. Disturbance of these targets, either directly by alkylation or as secondary results of disruptions to biochemical pathways, gives rise to a confusing array of cellular and tissue responses to HD. Recent data suggest that alteration of gene expression *(1)* and modification of cellular differentiation *(2)* are two pathways that could contribute to the toxic manifestations of HD exposure.

We used flow cytometry and monoclonal antibody (MAb) staining to determine whether expression of intracellular antigens thought to be associated with DNA damage and dysregulation of cell-cycle events could be affected by in vitro exposure of human epidermal keratinocytes (HEK) to HD. Since HEK are believed to be the in vitro equivalent to

From: *Toxicity Assessment Alternatives: Methods, Issues, Opportunities*
Edited by: H. Salem and S. A. Katz © Humana Press Inc., Totowa, NJ

Table 1
MAbs Used

Descriptor	Fluorotag[a]	Source	Clone	Target antigen
p53	Unconjug.	Sanbio	BP53.12	p53 nuclear antigen
	Unconjug.	Boehringer	Pab 122	
	PE	Pharmingen	G59-12	
	PE	Pharmingen	PAB 1801	
bcl2	FITC	DAKO	124	25-kDa bcl2 oncoprotein
PCNA	FITC	DAKO	PC10	36-kDa proliferating cell nuclear antigen
CK	FITC	B-Dickinson	CAM 5.2	Keratin 8 and 18
	FITC	DAKO	MNF116	Keratin 10, 17 and 18
EpitAg	FITC	DAKO	Ber-EP4	34- and 49-kDa surface antigens
EMA	FITC	DAKO	E-29	295- and 400-kDa surface antigen
CD62P	FITC	Pharmingen	AK4	140-kDa platelet antigen

[a]PE; phycoerythrin, FITC; fluorescein; and unconjug.; unconjugated antibody stained with second antibody (FITC conjugated rat antimouse).

skin basal epidermal cells and altered patterns of differentiation of basal cells might contribute to vesication, similar experiments were conducted using MAbs against HEK surface antigens related to their differentiation state.

METHODS

HEK were obtained as primary cultures from Clonetics, San Diego CA and maintained in serum-free keratinocyte growth medium (KGM). HD (>98% purity) was obtained from the US Army Edgewood Research, Development, and Engineering Center. Directly conjugated MAbs were purchased commercially from the following: Sanbio (Netherlands); Boehringer (Indianapolis, IN); Pharmingen (San Diego, CA); DAKO (Carpinter, CA); Becton Dickinson (San Jose, CA). and are described in Table 1.

HEK were grown in 75-cm^2 tissue-culture flask to 60–80% confluency, and then exposed to HD diluted in KGM to a final concentration of 100 μM. Media were not changed for the duration of the experiments. At the designated time-points, media were decanted, trypsin-EDTA was added for 5 min, and the cells were removed from the flasks by scraping. The cell suspension was mixed with trypsin-neutralizing solution, washed in KGM, and fixed with 1% formaldehyde for 15 min followed by 70% ethanol. Fixed cells were stored at –20°C until stained for cytometry.

Table 2
Effect of HD Exposure on HEK Antigen Expression 24 H Postexposure

HD conc.,	Change in antigen expression[a]						
μM	p53	bcl2	PCNA	CK	EpitAg	EMA	CD62P
10	+	−	+	+	+	NC	NC
50	+	−	+	+	+	NC	NC
100	+	−	+	+	+	NC	NC
200	++	−	++	+	+	NC	NC

[a]+, ++, increased expression; −, decreased expression; NC, no change.

Flow cytometric analyses were conducted on a Becton-Dickinson FACStar Plus cytometer using a 100 mW air-cooled argon laser at 488 nm.

RESULTS

Within 24 h of HD exposure in vitro, increased expression was detected for p53, PCNA, CK, and EpitAg (Table 2). Data not presented demonstrated that p53 was increased within 8 h of exposure. When p53 was increased, bcl2 expression was decreased. Expression of neither EMA nor the negative control CD62P was affected by HD exposure (Table 2).

DISCUSSION

Alterations of p53, bcl2, and PCNA expression are probably related to cell-cycle blockages generated by DNA-damaging effects of HD. Activation of p53 following DNA damage is believed to be an important step in generating the apoptotic death of damaged cells (3,4). The oncoprotein bcl2 blocks apoptosis and usually follows an activation pattern reciprocal to p53 (5). Increased p53 antigen expression may be related to induction of stress gene responses as reported by Schlager et al. (1). PCNA expression has been correlated with cyclin activity in HEK (6) and with DNA excision repair (7).

Increased expression of CK and EpitAg may signal a direct effect on HEK differentiation, which, in vivo, could alter the adhesion of basal keratinocytes to the basement membrane. The two CK antibodies used share reactivity with keratin 18, which is usually associated with skin appendages, not normal epidermis (8). The EpitAg is used to define normal and neoplastic cells of epithelial origin, but its upregulation in normal cells has not been reported.

Although no definitive associations can be made between the changes seen and alterations to the DNA or to differentiation status, these data support the continued utilization of immunodiagnostic procedures and flow cytometry of human cells exposed to HD. Future studies with cellular biochemical changes and altered patterns of gene regulation may provide the links for such associations.

REFERENCES

1. Schlager JJ, Smith WJ, Hart BW. Sulfur mustard (HD) stress gene induction in transformed Hep G2 cells. Proceedings of the 1996 Medical Defense Bioscience Review, US Army Medical Research Institute of Chemical Defense, APG, MD, 1996;2:1055–1061 (DTIC Accession # AD A321841).
2. Bernstein IA, Bernstam LI, Yang YH, Lin PP, Vaughan FL. Pseudo-epidermis: A model system for investigating molecular and cellular pathways of cutaneous epidermal toxicity from sulfur mustard. Proceedings of the 1993 Medical Defense Bioscience Review, USAMRICD, APG, MD 1993;1:97–104, Accession # AD A275667.
3. Kastan MB, Onyekwere O, Sidransky D, Vogelstein B, Craig R. Participation of p53 protein in the cellular response to DNA damage. Canc Res 1991;51:6304–6311.
4. Selivanova G, Wilman KG. p53: A cell cycle regulator activated by DNA damage. Adv Cancer Res 1995;66:143–180.
5. Cory S. Regulation of lymphocyte survival by the bcl-2 gene family. Annu Rev Immunol 1995;13:513–543.
6. Miyagawa S, Okada N, Takasaki Y, Iida T, Kitano Y, Yoshikawa K, et al. Expression of proliferating cell nuclear antigen/cyclin in human keratinocytes. J Invest Dermatol 1989;93:678–681.
7. Dietrich DR. Toxicological and pathological applications of proliferating cell nuclear antigen (PCNA), a novel endogenous marker for cell proliferation. Crit Rev Toxicol 1993;23:77–109.
8. Goddard MJ, Wilson B, Grant JW. Comparison of commercially available cytokeratin antibodies in normal and neoplastic adult epithelial and non-epithelial tissues. J Clin Pathol 1991;44:660–663.

18 Effect of Sulfur Mustard Exposure on Human Epidermal Keratinocyte Viability and Protein Content

William J. Smith, PhD, James A. Blank, PhD, Rebekah A. Starner, BSc, Ronald G. Menton, PhD, and Joy L. Harris

Contents

INTRODUCTION

Sulfur mustard (HD) is a bifunctional alkylating agent that has mutagenic, cytotoxic, and vesicating properties *(1–3)*. Although HD preferentially alkylates DNA, it is also known to modify RNA and proteins covalently *(4)*. DNA alkylation has been postulated to be the molecular mechanism that initiates a cascade of events terminating in vesication *(5)*. DNA alkylating agents, like HD, have been shown to cause unbalanced cell growth, a condition that occurs when cells exposed to cytotoxic drugs increase in cell volume, protein, and RNA content as cellular mass accumulates, but the cells fail to undergo cell division *(6,7)*. Depending on concentration, HD will produce different effects in vitro, ranging from inhibition of proliferation with unbalanced cell growth at lower concentrations to cytotoxicity at higher exposure levels

From: *Toxicity Assessment Alternatives: Methods, Issues, Opportunities*
Edited by: H. Salem and S. A. Katz © Humana Press Inc., Totowa, NJ

(4,8). With an inhibition of proliferation occurring with HD-exposed human epidermal keratinocytes (HEKs), measures of biochemical parameters taken from cultures at extended times postexposure must be standardized to account for differences in cell number. The primary objective of these studies was to assess the feasibility of using protein as a means of standardizing data across HD treatment groups.

MATERIALS AND METHODS

Tertiary cultures of HEKs were exposed to various concentrations of HD. At 0, 2, 24, 48, and 72 h following HD exposure, cultures were assessed for cell number, viability, and protein content.

Cell Cultures

Primary cultures of HEKs (Strain 2041) were received from Clonetics Corporation (San Diego, CA). Cells were clonally expanded in 25-cm^2 tissue-culture flasks using keratinocyte growth medium (Clonetics Corp.), and then subcultured as tertiary cultures in six-well tissue-culture plates. When cultures were 50–80% confluent, they were exposed to varying concentrations of HD. At 0, 2, 24, 48, and 72 h following HD exposure, cell supernatants were aspirated and placed into 15-mL conical centrifuge tubes. The adherent cells were detached from the plastic growth surface using trypsin-EDTA. The detached cells were combined with the supernatant and 3 mL of 1% fetal calf serum in RPMI 1640 medium (Gibco-BRL, Grand Island, NY). The samples were pelletized by centrifugation at 300g for 5 min. The supernatant was discarded, and the inside of the tube swabbed to remove adhering supernatant. The pellet was resuspended in 500 μL of Hank's Balanced Salt Solution (HBSS). Aliquots of the cell suspension were taken for cell enumeration, for viability determination, and for protein determination.

Cell Counts

Cell number was determined using a Coulter Model ZM (Coulter Electronics, Hialeah, FL) cell counter. The lower threshold was set at 7 μ using Coulter-sized microspheres.

Protein Assay

Protein content was determined by mixing cell-suspension aliquots with an equal volume of HBSS containing 2% Triton X-100. The samples were mixed well, and the protein content was determined using the BCA protein method (Pierce Chemical Company, Rockford, IL) with bovine serum albumin as the standard.

Viability Determinations

Cell suspensions (100 µL) were added to 900 µL of RPMI 1640 containing 30 µg of propidium iodide (PI). Viability was determined by measuring the number of PI-positive fluorescent cells out of 2000 cells evaluated. This was performed using a Becton Dickinson FACScan flow cytometer (San Jose, CA) equipped with an argon laser producing an incident beam of 488 nm.

Statistical Analysis

Results for each of three experimental runs were standardized using the time zero value for each parameter. An analysis of variance was performed on the pooled data to assess the effects of HD concentration and to estimate the components of variation for each data parameter. The analyses of variance were conducted using Proc Mixed, a mixed model analysis of variance procedure in SAS. Separate models were fitted to the data at each time-point for each data parameter. For each combination of time and data parameter, a hypothesis test was conducted to compare the average of each HD-exposed group to that of the control group.

RESULTS

Figures 1–5 illustrate data parameters that have been standardized to the time zero value as a function of both HD concentration and time following HD exposure. Data points plotted are the average of three experimental runs, with each experiment consisting of a minimum of two observations. The descriptive statistics for the data presented in the figures are presented in Table 1. As shown in Fig. 1, 13 μM HD had little effect on total culture protein relative to controls. The 72-h protein value was significantly ($p < 0.05$) less than the respective time control value. The three highest HD concentrations caused a significant ($p < 0.05$) depression in total protein that was first apparent at 24 h following exposure. Although there appeared to be some increase in protein content of cultures exposed to 62 and 101 μM HD from 24 to 72 h, no recovery was evident in cultures exposed to 171 μM HD.

Figure 2 illustrates the effect of HD on total cell number. The three highest HD concentrations had significant ($p < 0.05$) inhibitory effects on cellular proliferation by 24 h of exposure, whereas the effect of the lowest concentration was not significant until 48 h. The effect of HD on cell viability is shown in Fig. 3. Cytotoxicity was observed in cultures exposed to 171 μM HD, but was not observed at the lower HD concentrations. This effect was significant by 24 h of exposure and appeared

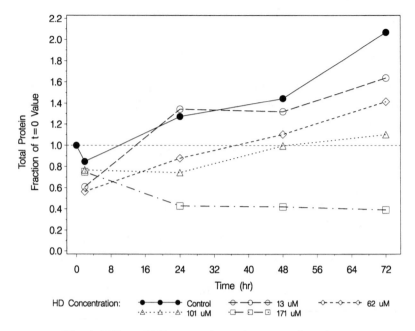

Fig. 1. Effect of HD on total protein content in cultures.

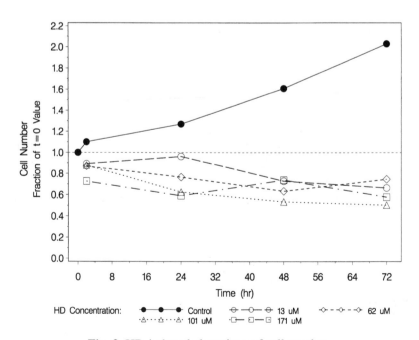

Fig. 2. HD-induced alterations of cell number.

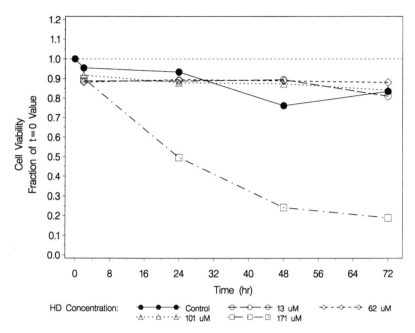

Fig. 3. Effect of HD on cellular viability measured by propidium iodide exclusion.

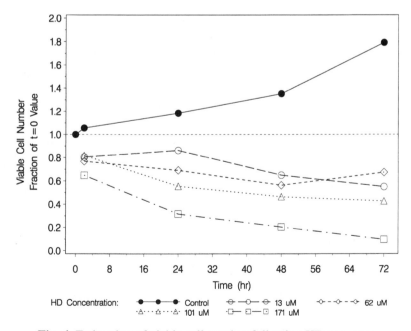

Fig. 4. Estimation of viable cell number following HD exposure.

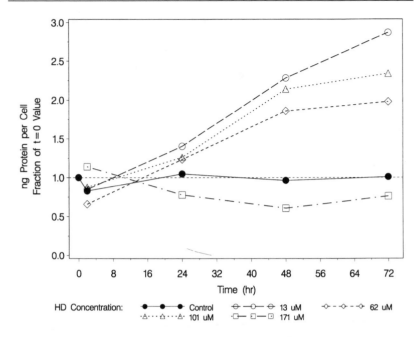

Fig. 5. Estimation of the amount of prtein per cell for each HD exposure.

to increase with time. Although HD exposure completely arrests cellular proliferation, only 171 μM HD produced significant ($p < 0.05$) cytotoxicity. Data for viable cell number obtained by multiplying total cell number by the fraction of viable cells are presented in Fig. 4. These data are similar to the total cell count data with the exception of the 171 μM HD-exposed groups, which are markedly lower owing to the cytotoxicity occurring at this concentration.

Figure 5 presents data for protein values normalized to cell number. The three lowest concentrations of HD increase the amount of protein per cell, which appears elevated by 24 h, but is not statistically significant until 48 h. The amount of protein per cell tended to increase as a function of time following HD exposure, except at 171 μM. The highest HD concentration, 171 μM, did not significantly ($p < 0.05$) affect the amount of protein per cell.

DISCUSSION

HD is a bifunctional alkylating agent that produces antiproliferative and cytotoxic effects on cells. Although HD alkylates DNA, RNA, and protein, DNA crosslinks and strand breaks are thought to be the primary insult responsible for cytotoxicity *(5)*. DNA alkylation by HD inhibits proliferation by causing cell-cycle blocks at the G1-S and G2-M boundaries with vesicating doses (>50–100 μM or higher), causing a G1-S block, and approx 10-fold lower HD concentrations, causing a G2-M block *(9)*.

In these studies, the effect of HD exposure on cellular protein levels was examined to assess the usefulness of protein as a measure for normalizing biochemical measures made on cultures where inhibition of cellular proliferation may be occurring. All HD concentrations inhibited cellular proliferation (Fig. 2); however, cells exposed to the three lowest HD concentrations (13, 62, and 101 μM) did not exhibit cytotoxicity and had elevated levels of protein per cell relative to controls (Fig. 5). This effect was significant by 48 h and was the highest at the 13 μM HD exposure (2.3-fold of control) and somewhat lower at the 62- and 101-μM exposures (1.9- and 2.1-fold of control, respectively). These data are consistent with the cell-cycle data of Smith et al. *(9)*, which indicate that a G2-M cell-cycle block should be occurring in this approximate concentration range. Information for other alkylating agents indicates that cells with G2-M blocks continue to synthesize RNA and protein, and increase cell volume without cellular replication occurring *(10)*. These data are also consistent with the data of Schlager et al. *(11)*, which demonstrated the expression of genes induced by cellular stress at HD concentrations that are not cytotoxic.

In contrast, the amount of protein per cell at the 171-μM HD concentration was not significantly different from controls (Fig. 5). At this HD concentration, there was no apparent recovery of protein synthesis (Fig. 1), and cytotoxicity was observed within 24 h of exposure (Fig. 3). Results at this exposure level are markedly different from those for the 101-μM HD group. Data from Smith et al. *(9)* indicate that this exposure level may be consistent with a G1-S block and would be considered at the vesicating level. These data are consistent with the findings of Mol and deVries-VandeRuit *(12)* in which HD concentrations in the vesicating range inhibited DNA replication and also inhibited protein synthesis. These data are also interesting with respect to previous findings of Martens *(13)*, which indicate a shift in the cellular energy source away from glucose at HD concentrations starting at approx 70 μM. It is possible that protein synthesis is being sacrificed or that enhanced protein catabolism is occurring in the terminal efforts of a cell to sustain cellular energy supplies.

Owing to the variable concentration- and time-dependent effects of HD on cellular proliferation and cellular metabolism, protein does not appear to be a suitable means of standardizing biochemical data for the human epidermal keratinocytes, particularly beyond 24 h of exposure.

These data are interesting in that marked differences exist in the cellular protein levels and viability between the 101- and the 171-μM HD exposure groups, and these differences seem to occur in the HD concentration range reported to cause vesication (50–100 μM or higher). If cessation of protein synthesis is an event associated with vesicating doses of HD, as suggested by Mol and deVries-VandeRuit *(12)*, then the biochemical events leading to this shutdown may provide insight into the development of a new therapeutic strategy to minimize HD-induced dermal toxicity.

REFERENCES

1. Cappizzi RL, Smith WJ, Field RJ, Papirmeister B. A host-mediated assay for chemical mutagens using the L5178Y/asn(-) murine leukemia. Mutat Res 1973;21:6.
2. Rozmiarek J, Cappizzi RL, Papirmeister B, Furman WH, Smith WJ. Mutagenic activity in somatic and germ cells following chronic inhalation of sulfur mustard. Mutat Res 1973;21:13.
3. Smith WJ, Sanders KM, Gross CL, Meier HL. Flow cytometric assessment of the effects of alkylation on viability, cell cycle, and DNA structure in human lymphocytes. Cytometry Suppl 1988;2:21.
4. Roberts JJ, Brent TP, Crathorn AR. Evidence for the inactivation and repair of the mammalian DNA template after alkylation by mustard gas and half mustard gas. Eur J Cancer 1971;7:515–524.
5. Papirmeister B, Gross CL, Meier HL, Petrali JP, Johnson JB. Molecular basis for mustard-induced vesication. Fundam App Toxicol 1985;5:S134–S139.
6. Ross DW. Unbalanced cell growth and increased protein synthesis induced by chemotherapeutic agents. Blood Cell 1983;9:57–68.
7. Cohen LS, Studzinski GP. Correlation between cell enlargement and nucleic acid and protein content of HeLa cells in unbalanced growth produced by inhibitors of DNA synthesis. J Cell Physiol 1967;69:331–340.
8. Smith WJ, Gross CL, Chan P, Meier HL. The use of human epidermal keratinocytes in culture as a model for studying the biochemical mechanisms of sulfur mustard toxicity. Cell Biol Toxicol 1990;6:285–291.
9. Smith WJ, Sanders KM, Ruddle SE, Gross CL. Cytometric analysis of DNA changes induced by sulfur mustard. J Toxicol Cutaneous Ocular Toxicol 1993;12: 343–353.
10. Calabresi P, Chabner BA. Chemotherapy of neoplastic diseases. In: Gilman A, Rall T, Nies A, Taylor P, eds. Goodman and Gilman's The Pharmacological Basis of Therapeutics, 8th ed. Pergamon, New York, 1990.
11. Schlager J, Smith WJ, Hart BW. Sulfur mustard (HD) stress gene induction in transformed HEP G2 cells. The Toxicologist 1996;30:328.
12. Mol MAE, deVries-VandeRuit A-MBC. Concentration and time-related effects of sulphur mustard on human epidermal keratinocyte function. Toxicol In Vitro 1992;6:235–251.
13. Martens ME. Biochemical studies of sulfur mustard-induced injury. Proc 4th Symposium on Protection Against Chemical Warfare Agents, 1992, pp. 325–331.

19 The Use of In Vitro Systems to Define Therapeutic Approaches to Cutaneous Injury by Sulfur Mustard

William J. Smith, PhD, Margaret E. Martens, PhD, Clark L. Gross, MS, Offie E. Clark, BS, Fred M. Cowan, BS, and Jeffrey J. Yourick, PhD

CONTENTS

INTRODUCTION

Sulfur mustard (HD) is an alkylating agent that has been shown to have mutagenic, cytotoxic, and vesicating properties. Its use in combat situations has resulted in lethal, incapacitating, and disfiguring injuries. The principal incapacitating injuries come from the vesicating capacity of HD, i.e., production of skin blisters *(1)*. Despite decades of medical research, the mechanism by which HD induces vesication is not known, and no effective antidotes are currently available. The studies in this chapter utilize flow cytometric, biochemical, and histopathological analyses of human and animal cells and tissues for the toxicologic assessment of HD-induced damage. These techniques allowed a unique

From: *Toxicity Assessment Alternatives: Methods, Issues, Opportunities*
Edited by: H. Salem and S. A. Katz © Humana Press Inc., Totowa, NJ

series of experiments to be conducted that defined levels of sensitivity in human cells to both the cytotoxic and genotoxic effects of HD. These studies, in turn, have provided data that are relevant to the development of therapeutic intervention in the human pathology produced by HD.

METHODS

Lymphocyte Isolation

Human peripheral blood lymphocytes (PBL) were isolated from whole blood obtained by venipuncture from volunteers under an approved human use protocol by density centrifugation through histopaque (d = 1.077, Sigma, St. Louis, MO). The isolated PBL were resuspended in RPMI-1640 with 5% fetal bovine serum (RPMI-FBS).

Epithelial Cell Cultures

Human epithelial keratinocytes (HEK) were grown in keratinocyte growth medium (KGM) under conditions defined by the manufacturer (Clonetics, San Diego, CA). The human epithelial tumor cell line, HeLa, was grown in RPMI-1640 with 5% fetal bovine serum (Sigma). All culture conditions were described in Smith et al. *(2)*.

Agent Exposures

Hairless guinea pigs were exposed cutaneously to HD vapor for 8 min through the use of Edgewood vapor cups as described in Yourick et al. *(3)*. The investigators adhered to "Guide for the Care and Use of Laboratory Animals" NIH Publication No 85-23, revised in 1985. For in vitro exposures of PBL, HeLa, or HEK, HD was dissolved in aqueous tissue-culture media and added to the cells at the desired final concentrations.

Flow Cytometry

Propidium iodide (PI) in RPMI medium was used for assessment of cellular viability on a Becton-Dickinson FACStar Plus cytometer (BDIS, San Jose, CA). A trypsin-detergent procedure for intercalation of PI into cellular DNA was used for DNA analysis *(4)*.

Protease Assay

A chromogenic peptide substrate assay using Chromozym substrates (Boehringer Mannheim, Indianapolis, IN) as described in Cowan et al. *(5)* was used.

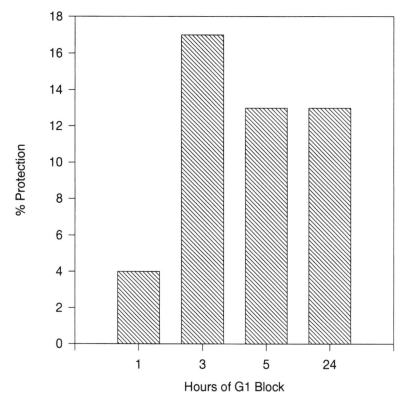

Fig. 1. Mimosine protection of HeLa cell viability following HD.

RESULTS

Previous reports from our laboratory have established that proliferating PBL are more sensitive to the cytotoxicity of HD than are quiesent PBL *(6)*. Furthermore, we showed that cells in the S phase of the cell cycle are more sensitive than cells in G0 or G1. Although we initially reported that HD had direct inhibitory effects on cell-cycle progression by blocking cells at the G1/S interface *(6)*, we subsequently found that the cell-cycle blocking patterns of HD were concentration-dependent *(4)*. These observations led us to explore the protective efficacy of cell-cycle inhibitors on HD cytotoxicity. Figure 1 shows that the reversible G1 inhibitor mimosine, when used to hold HD-exposed cells in G1 for varying periods of time postexposure, can provide protection against loss of cell viability.

It has long been held that HD produces toxicity by direct alkylation of critical cellular macromolecules. We therefore evaluated the possibil-

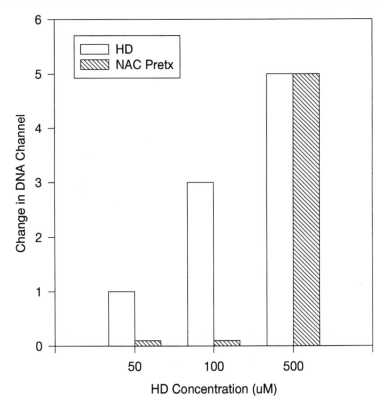

Fig. 2. Alteration of DNA stainability by propidium iodide in human PBL follow-ing HD exposure in the presence or absence of N-acetyl-L-cysteine (10 m*M*).

ity of enhancing intracellular concentrations of the protective scavenger glutathione *(7)*. *N*-acetyl-cysteine (NAC), a prodrug of glutathione, provided a moderate level of protection against the loss of viability by PBL exposed in vitro to HD. In addition, as shown in Fig. 2 pretreatment with NAC abrogates the concentration-dependent DNA structural changes in HD-exposed PBL.

One of the most consistent observations in cells and tissues exposed to HD is a time- and concentration-dependent loss of cellular NAD+ *(8)*. This loss of NAD+ is caused by activation of the nuclear enzyme poly(ADP-ribose) polymerase (PARP), which uses NAD+ as a sub-strate. Inhibitors of PARP have been the leading candidates for vesicant countermeasures, and niacinamide is a prototypic PARP inhibitor *(9)*. Figure 3 demonstrates the efficacy of niacinamide in ameliorating microvesical formation in the hairless guinea pig following cutaneous exposure to vapor HD.

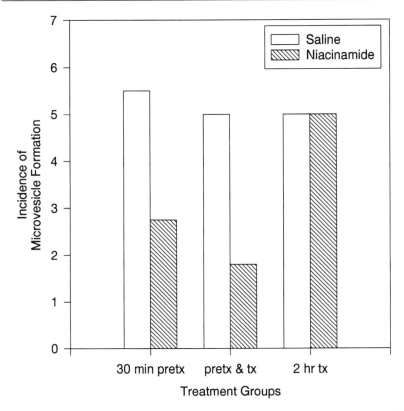

Fig. 3. Skin biopsies from animals exposed to 8 munte cutaneous vapor HD with or without niacinamide as a pre- and/or post-exposure treatment.

Since the tissue injury elicited by HD involves a reproducible separation in the subbasallar region of the skin, a role for proteolytic degradation of adhesion molecules located at the epidermal–dermal junction has been proposed *(1)*. We have demonstrated proteolytic induction in PBL *(4)*, epithelial cells *(10)*, and hairless guinea pig skin biopsies *(11,12)* following exposures to HD. Figure 4 demonstrates the efficacy of NAC, niacinamide, and dexamethasone in modulating the proteolysis in HD-exposed PBL. In addition, two compounds capable of serving as anti-inflammatory agents, phenidone and hydroxyurea, were shown to reduce the HD-increased proteolysis in hairless guinea pig skin *(13)*.

DISCUSSION

Army Science and Technology Objective (STO) V.A—"Medical Countermeasures Against Vesicant Agents" calls for development of

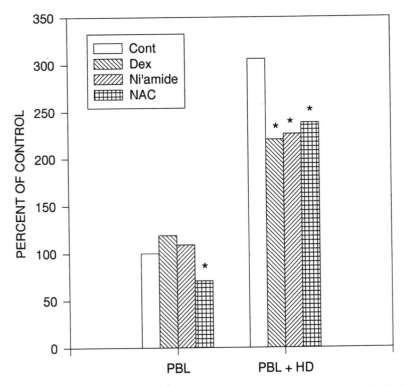

Fig. 4. Inhibition of HD-induced proteolysis in human PBL treated with niacinamide (1 mM), dexamethasone (0.1 μM), or N-acetyl-L-cysteine (10 mM).

strategies for prophylaxis, pretreatment, and antidote therapy that will provide significant protection against vesicant injury and to demonstrate, by FY00, safety and efficacy of a candidate medical countermeasure sufficient for milestone 0 transition. The data presented in this chapter lead to the presentation of several such strategies:

1. With DNA as a critical cellular target of alkylation by mustards, regulators of cell-cycle progression, such as mimosine, may find endogenous DNA repair capabilities to minimize acute and chronic tissue damage.
2. Intracellular scavengers, such as glutathione, might be exploited to serve as alternative alkylation sites, thereby sparing critical cellular macromolecules from damage.
3. Inhibitor application as local topical formulations to allow the damaged epithelial tissue to utilize PARP, as seen with niacinamide, can lower the incidence of microblister formation.
4. Characterization of the proteolytic response to HD will lead to definition of a pathway or cascade that can be interdicted by specific antiproteases.

Table 1
Sulfur Mustard Pathology—Potential Pharmacological Interventions

Biochemical damage	Compound category	Example
DNA alkylation	Intracellular scavengers	N-acetyl cysteine
DNA strand breaks	Cell-cycle inhibitors	Mimosine
PARP activation	PARP inhibitors	Niacinamide
Disruption of calcium	Calcium modulators	BAPTA
Proteolytic activation	Protease inhibitors	AEBSF
Inflammation	Anti-inflammatories	Phenidone

The results in this chapter have generated four therapeutic approaches by vesicant countermeasures. Two other approaches being studied at the US Army Medical Research Institute of Chemical Defense, calcium modulation *(14)* and anti-inflammatory drugs *(15,16)*, bring the total strategies available at this time to six (Table 1). In the next few years, there will be movement of the lead candidates from one or more of these strategies to advanced drug development, so that our goal of "Research for the Soldier" will be fully met.

ACKNOWLEDGMENTS

The authors wish to thank Shannon Ruddle, Eilleen Emison, Jennifer VanBergen, James Caulfield, Michael Sanders, Yolanda Gales, Katherine Garwood, and Joy Innace for their excellent technical assistance. This work was supported under Science and Technology Objective (STO) V.A.—"Medical Countermeasures Against Vesicant Agents."

REFERENCES

1. Papirmeister B, Feister AJ, Robinson SI, Ford RD. Medical Defense Against Mustard Gas: Toxic Mechanisms and Pharmacological Implications, CRC, Boca Raton, FL, 1991.
2. Smith WJ, Gross CL, Chan P, Meier HL. The use of human epidermal keratinocytes. In: Culture is a Model for Studying the Biochemical Mechanisms of Sulfur Mustard Toxicity. Cell Biol Toxicol 1990;6:285–291.
3. Yourick JJ, Clark CR, Mitcheltree L. Niacinamide pretreatment reduces microvesicle formation in hairless guinea pigs cutaneously exposed to sulfur mustard. Fundam Appl Toxicol 1991;17:533–542.
4. Smith WJ, Sanders KM, Ruddle SE, Gross CL. Cytometric analysis of DNA changes induced by sulfur mustard. J Toxicol—Cutaneous Ocular Toxicol 1993; 12:343–353.
5. Cowan FM, Broomfield CA, Smith WJ. Effect of sulfur mustard exposure on protease activity in human peripheral blood lymphocytes. Cell Biol Toxicol 1991;7: 239–248.

6. Smith WJ, Sanders KM, Gales YA, Gross CL. Flow cytometric analysis of toxicity by vesicating agents in human cells *in vitro*. J Toxicol—Cutaneous Ocular Toxicol 1991;10(1):33–42.

7. Gross CL, Innace JK, Hovatter RC, Meier HL, Smith WJ. Biochemical manipulation of intracellular glutathione levels influences cytotoxicity to isolated human lymphocytes by sulfur mustard. Cell Biol Toxicol 1993;9:259–268.

8. Meier HL, Gross HL, Papirmeister B. 2,2'-dichlorodiethyl sulfide (sulfur mustard) decreases NAD+ levels in human leukocytes. Toxicol Lett 1987;39:109–122.

9. Meier HL, Johnson JB. The determination and prevention of cytotoxic effects induced in human lymphocytes by the alkylating agent 2,2'-dichlorodiethyl sulfide (sulfur mustard, HD). Toxicol Appl Pharmacol 1992;113:234–239.

10. Cowan FM, Broomfield CA, Smith WJ. Increased proteolytic activity in human epithelial cells following exposure to sulfur mustard. Proceedings of the ERDEC Scientific Conference on Chemical and Biological Defense Research, US Army Edgewood Research, Development and Engineering Center, APG, MD, 1995.

11. Cowan FM, Yourick JJ, Hurst CG, Broomfield CA, Smith WJ. Sulfur mustard-increased proteolysis following in vitro and in vivo exposures. Cell Biol Toxicol 1993;9:253–262.

12. Cowan FM, Bongiovanni R, Broomfield CA, Yourick JJ, Smith WJ. Sulfur mustard-increased elastase-like activity in homogenates of hairless guinea pig skin. J Toxicol—Cutaneous Ocular Toxicol 1994;13:221–229.

13. Cowan FM, Bongiovanni R, Broomfield CA, Schulz SM, Smith WJ. Phenidone and hydroxyurea reduce sulfur mustard-increased proteolysis in hairless guinea pig skin. J Toxicol—Cutaneous Ocular Toxicol 1995;14:265–272.

14. Ray R, Benton BJ, Anderson DR, Byers SL, Petrali JP. Calcium chelator (BAPTA) as a prospective antidote against mustard gas. Proceedings of the 20th Army Science Conference, 1996.

15. Cowan FM, Broomfield CA. Putative roles of inflammation in the dermatopathology of sulfur mustard. Cell Biol Toxicol 1993;9:201–214.

16. Casillas RP, Smith KJ, Lee RB, Castrejon LR, Stemler FW. Effect of topically applied drugs against HD-induced cutaneous injury in the mouse ear edema model. Proceedings of the 1996 Medical Defense Bioscience Review, US Army Medical Research Institute of Chemical Defense, APG, MD, 1996.

20 Effects of Poly (ADP-Ribose) Polymerase Inhibitors on the Sulfur Mustard-Induced Disruption of the Higher-Order Nuclear Structure of Human Lymphocytes

Henry L. Meier, PhD
and Charles B. Millard, PhD

CONTENTS

INTRODUCTION
METHODS
RESULTS
DISCUSSION
REFERENCES

INTRODUCTION

Sulfur mustard (HD) is a potent vesicant that can cause severe lesions to skin, lung, and eyes *(1)*. To develop therapeutic pretreatment or treatment regimens to prevent HD-initiated damage, a better understanding of the mechanisms of action of HD is required. Based on the initial findings by Herriott and Price *(2)*, DNA was implicated as an important target in causing the cellular effects of HD. Berger et al. *(3)* proposed a hypothesis for the mechanism of cell death owing to exposure to alkylating agents, which was dependent on alkylation of the cell's DNA. The alkylation of the DNA results in DNA strand breaks, which cause activation of the nuclear enzyme poly (ADP-ribose) polymerase (PARP). Active PARP could deplete the cell of nicotinamide-adenine dinucle-

From: *Toxicity Assessment Alternatives: Methods, Issues, Opportunities*
Edited by: H. Salem and S. A. Katz © Humana Press Inc., Totowa, NJ

213

otide (NAD). The depletion of NAD would inhibit glycolysis and result in a loss of adenosine triphosphate (ATP). The ATP is needed as the major source of energy required for cell survival. Berger's hypothesis has been extensively evaluated using the alkylator HD. It has been demonstrated in peripherial blood lymphocytes (PBLs) that HD lowers cell viability *(4)*, NAD *(5)*, and ATP *(6)* levels of the exposed cells. Protection against these HD-initiated losses could be shown using poly (ADP-ribose) polymerase inhibitors (PARPIs). Recent studies examined the effects of HD on Berger's proposed primary target, the nucleus, and the effects of PARPIs were investigated. The most abundant nuclear proteins, histones, show altered solubility in PBLs exposed to HD. The structure of at least one histone, histone H2B, has been changed by what appears to be proteolytic cleavage *(7)*. PARPIs appeared to have minimal effect on HD-induced changes in histones. This work attempts to address the effect of HD on DNA directly. The effects of HD on the DNA in PBLs were determined by both agarose-gel electrophoresis and flow cytometry. HD caused a concentration and time-dependent fragmentation of the DNA in PBLs. When PARPIs were present in the PBL incubation mixture, they did not prevent the DNA cleavage initiated by HD, but they did alter the resulting cleavage patterns.

METHODS

Isolation and Exposure of PBLs

Blood (≤200 mL) was drawn from normal human volunteers under an approved human-use protocol. PBLs were isolated from blood by centrifugation on a Percoll gradient (density = 1.080 at 20°C) as previously described *(4)*. Cell counts were obtained using a hemacytometer. In 96-well plates, 10^6 cells/well were placed for viability and DNA peak shift experiments, and in 24-well plates, $10-15 \times 10^6$ cells/well were placed for DNA extraction. The cells, buffer (RPMI 1640M medium), and the test compound were added to the wells of tissue-culture plates 15 min before the appropriate volume of HD was added. The plates were placed in a 37°C CO_2 incubator for the indicated time.

Determination of PBLs Viability

PBLs viability was determined by measuring the ability of the PBLs to exclude propidium iodide (PI) from each individual cell. PBLs were removed from the plate, added to a tube containing 50 µL of PI, and allowed to incubate at 22°C for 3 min. The cells were then assayed for PI staining using a Becton Dickinson FACSort (San Jose, CA).

DNA Extraction and Electrophoresis

The cells were removed from the plates and processed using the G Nome protocol kit (Bio 101, Inc., La Jolla, CA). Total genomic DNA was purified using protease K, RNAse, and a differential salt extraction protocol, followed by ethanol precipitation overnight at –10°C. Solubilized DNA in TE buffer was evaluated by electrophoresis using 1–3% (w/v) agarose gels (7).

RESULTS

Effects of Cytotoxicity on Genomic DNA in PBLs

PBLs were exposed to HD, Lewisite, which is another powerful vesicating agent, or heat as cytotoxic stimuli, and genomic DNA patterns were subsequently studied 24 h later. Lewisite was the most cytotoxic of the stimuli (66% dead), but on agarose gels, there was no detectable shift in migration of the DNA from the control cells (<3% dead). Heating the PBLs to 55°C for 30 min, and continuing the incubation at 37°C for 24 h (41% dead) did not change the DNA pattern on agarose gels from that of controls. However, the exposure of the PBLs to 3×10^{-4} M HD (40% dead) caused fragmentation of the DNA as measured by both an increase in the distance the genomic DNA migrated into the gels and by a widening of the band.

The HD Concentration Dependence of the Fragmentation Pattern Shift

PBLs were exposed to HD (10^{-6}–$10^{-3}M$) to determine whether the fragmentation of genomic DNA was concentration-dependent (Fig. 1). Changes in the genomic DNA patterns from PBLs 24 h after exposure were detected at HD concentrations as low as 3×10^{-6} M. As the concentration of HD was increased, the shift in the DNA pattern changed from slight tailing to heavy tailing into the gel. At the highest HD concentrations studied, DNA appeared as a dense band that migrated farthest into the gel (Fig. 1).

The Concentration Dependence of the Shift in the Binding of PI Induced by HD

PBLs were exposed to HD at various concentrations, and at 24 h postexposure, their DNA was incubated with PI. The DNA changes were

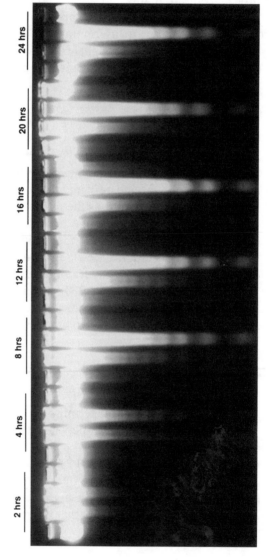

Fig. 1. Electrophoresis (2.5% agarose) of total genomic DNA extracted using the Gnome Kit (Bio 101) from PBLs exposed to increasing concentrations of HD. Lanes 1 and 12 are the DNA extracted form unexposed control PBLs. Lanes 2–11 are DNA isolated from PBLs exposed to the following HD concentrations, respectively: 10^{-3}; 6×10^{-4}; 3×10^{-4}; 10^{-4}; 6×10^{-5}; 3×10^{-5}; 10^{-5}; 6×10^{-6}; 3×10^{-6}; and 10^{-6}.

studied using the intensity of the binding of PI to the genomic DNA in PBLs as measured by flow cytometry. There was a shift to the right of the peak channel fluorescence, which was proportional to the concentration of HD to which the cells were exposed. The shift in the fluorescence peak was detected at concentrations as low as $1 \times 10^{-5} M$ HD (data not shown).

Time Dependence of HD-Initiated Fragmentation of Human PBLs Genomic DNA

PBLs were exposed to $3 \times 10^{-4} M$ HD at time zero. At 2, 4, 8, 12, 16, 20, and 24 h after exposure, a small volume of the control or HD-exposed cells was removed and assayed for peak fluorescence shift and DNA pattern. The shift in the fluorescence measured by flow cytometry began as early as 2 h post-HD exposure and shifted further to the right with time. The DNA that was extracted from the HD-exposed cells and underwent electrophoresis demonstrated some fragmentation as early as 2 h post-HD exposure. The fragmentation appeared to increase over the first 12 h post-HD exposure, resulting in increased migration and tailing of the DNA band into the gel. This DNA tail appeared to consist of a ladder of decreasing size fragments. Beginning between 12 and 16 h post-HD exposure, the DNA fragmentation pattern changed. The DNA tail, which was lengthened during the first 12 h post-HD exposure, now began to decrease in length, and the ladder pattern seemed to disappear. By 24 h post-HD exposure, the ladder pattern completely disappeared, and the main band of the DNA increased its migration into the gel.

Change in DNA Fragmentation Pattern as a Result of the Addition of PARPI

PBLs were exposed to buffer alone, buffer with HD, buffer with PARPI, or buffer with PARPI and HD. Then incubation times were varied so that the DNA was extracted at 2, 4, 6, 12, 16, 20, or 24 h post-HD exposure. The cells incubated in buffer alone or with PARPI showed for all time-points a single narrow band of DNA that migrated a similar distance in the gel. The DNA patterns changed with time for both the cells incubated with HD and the cells incubated with PARPI and HD. The initial pattern observed at 2 h for the HD alone and with PARPI and HD was a band wider than control that migrated with a tail further into the gel. From 4 to 12 h post-HD exposure, both the cells with HD alone and those with HD and PARPI developed tails with a ladder-type structure whose length increased with time. As the incubation increased from 12 to 24 h, the gel patterns of HD again changed so that the migration of the tail into the gel decreased with time and the ladder-like patterns decreased with time. By 24 h, the DNA pattern of the HD-exposed cells degenerated to a wide band with no tailing of a ladder. The pattern of DNA from cells incubated with PARPI and HD showed with time an increase in the length of the tailing and an increase in ladder formation. During the entire time period, the length of the tailing of DNA from cells exposed to HD was shorter than that observed for the DNA of cells incubated with PARPI and HD. Though the DNA of cells incubated with PARPI and HD showed extensive DNA fragmentation, the loss of viability as measured by PI incorporation was low especially compared to cells incubated with HD alone (8). The shift in the peak channel fluorescence for cells incubated with PARPI and HD was also less than that observed in the cells incubated with HD alone.

The Effect of Delaying the Addition of PARPI on the DNA Changes

HD was added to cell incubation mixture at time zero. A PARPI was added to the mixture at the indicated times, and the incubation continued for 24 h post-HD exposure before the DNA extraction. The DNA pattern (Fig. 2) of control was a narrow band just a short distance into the gel, as seen previously. DNA from cells exposed to HD without PARPI presented as a wider band with a short tail, which migrated further into the gel than that from the control. However, the patterns seen in the gel of the DNA of cells to which HD was added at time zero and PARPI at indicated times varied with the time of PARPI addition. The pattern of the DNA from the cells in the mixture to which the PARPI was added at either an hour before HD addition or during the first 2 h post-HD addition demonstrated a loss of the higher bands of DNA and the formation of a distinct ladder pattern. However, when the PARPI addition was delayed 4 h post-HD exposure, the lower portion of the ladder pattern appeared to decrease, and when it was added 8 h or later post-HD exposure, the ladder pattern did not appear to form. The later the PARPI was added to the incubation mixture, the more of the tail that was lost. The protection of viability by PARPI addition in PBLs exposed to HD decreased as the time of addition was delayed. Also the partial inhibition of the peak fluorescence right shift seen in cell DNA analyzed by flow cytometry decreased with the increase in the delay. Thus, the later the PARPI was added to the cells, the more PI was incorporated in the DNA of HD-exposed cells.

HD (M) -->

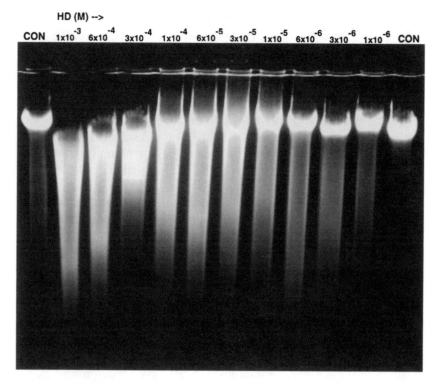

Fig. 2. Delayed addition of PARPI determines how the genomic DNA is fragmented. HD (3×10^{-4} M) is given to cells at time 0. The PARPI ICD-2250 is given at the indicated times, and the cells are incubated for 24 h post-HD exposure. If the PARPI is added as late as 8 h post-HD exposure, then it fails to stop the DNA fragmentation at the ladder stage.

DISCUSSION

To provide the soldier with an effective medical countermeasure to prevent HD-induced vesication, it is essential to understand the biochemical changes initiated by HD. It was known that HD alkylated DNA. Until now, the mechanism of DNA damage had not been elucidated. The work outlined in this chapter not only indicates what appears to be the mechanism of DNA damage, but also demonstrates the results of the damage. Based on these finding, there is now a better understanding of how to approach the development of an anti-HD treatment.

HD exposure resulted in cleavage of nuclear DNA in PBLs. Though there appears to be little difference between individual DNA fragmentation patterns initiated by HD and the degree of peak fluorescence shifting to the right, significant conclusions can be drawn about the effects of HD on DNA. The cleavage of the DNA appears to be the result of a specific mechanism initiated by alkylation of the DNA as a result of exposure to HD and not the result of cell death, nor is fragmentation of DNA a characteristic action of vesicating agents, since exposure to Lewisite, a potent vesicating agent and cytotoxic compound, does not result in any detectable fragmentation of DNA. Based on an increase in the incorporation of PI in the DNA of HD (10^{-3} and 10^{-5} M) exposed PBLs, it has been concluded that HD causes a concentration-dependent disruption of the structure of the nucleus. This increase in PI incorporation is measured by a shift to the right of the fluorescence peak channel, which appears to indicate an unfolding of DNA to increase accessibility of DNA for PI binding. The higher the concentration of HD in the exposure, the further the peak channel is shifted to the right, suggesting that higher concentrations of HD lead to greater disruptions of DNA structure. The study of DNA fragmentation by agarose gels also appears to support this hypothesis. The higher the HD exposure, the more fragmentation is observed. This method of determining HD effects on DNA appears to be more sensitive than the peak channel shift, since even at concentrations as low as 10^{-6} M HD, some fragmentation (tailing into the gel) is observed at 24 h. However, the fluorescence peak channel shift can be utilized to develop an assay for determining efficacy of anti-HD treatment regimens, since it appears to measure a quantitative change in DNA structure, which is dependent both on the time after and the concentration of HD exposure.

When other biological effects of HD on PBLs were investigated (decreases in viability, NAD levels, and ATP levels), it was determined that these HD-initiated alterations could be blocked or inhibited by PARPI. The amount of protection conferred to the PBLs against HD-initiated changes appeared to be proportional to the ability of the drugs to inhibit PARPI (4). Therefore, these PARPIs were studied to determine whether they protected the DNA from HD-initiated fragmentation of the DNA. However, PARPIs only partially block the right shift in the PI peak fluorescence shift. This would tend to indicate that the fragmentation of the DNA as a result of HD exposure was altered, but it was not prevented. This is supported by the fragmentation patterns observed on agarose gels. The PARPI caused an alteration of the DNA pattern from that seen in necrotic lesions to a DNA fragmentation pattern characteristic of the ladder pattern seen in apoptotic cell death (9). The DNA in the HD-exposed cells in the presence of PARPIs appears to be extensively fragmented. However, these cells were not dead as defined by the exclusion of PI. Thus, it appears that the PARPIs not only prevent "cell death" and the loss of metabolic function, but also alter the mechanism of DNA cleavage. The PARPIs appear to prevent the breakdown of the cell membrane and the loss of metabolic function while permitting an apoptotic fragmentation to occur in the nuclei. This would indicate that the PBLs that are exposed to HD in the presence of PARPIs are metabolically viable, but reproductively terminated cells. When a time-course of HD-initiated DNA fragmentation was analyzed on agarose gels, the initial fragmentation that occurred during the first 2–12 h post-HD exposure appeared to be a ladder pattern similar to that observed during apoptotic changes. However, by 16 h post-HD exposure, the fragmentation pattern lost its ladder-type structure and the length of the tailing decreased. Thus, it appears that two independent DNA fragmentation mechanisms may be involved in HD-initiated DNA fragmentation. Initially, the mechanism that produces ladder-type structures prevails, but after awhile, the ladders disappear and the wide band indicative of necrotic-type DNA damage predominates.

There are candidate antivesicant compounds that can block the necrotic fragmentation and prevent cell death by this mechanism. Based on this study, it has been determined that along with PARPI, which prevent necrotic DNA cleavage, inhibitors of apoptosis-like changes must be added to an anti-HD regimen so that the cells will not only maintain viability, but also retain function. The combination of these two components in a candidate anti-HD therapeutic regimen should not only prevent HD cytotoxicity, but also enable the HD-damaged cells to maintain the integrity of their DNA, and perhaps permit the cells to repair the HD-initiated damage. This may assist some of the cells with HD-damaged DNA to reproduce and to maintain normal function.

REFERENCES

1. McNamara BP. Medical Aspects of Chemical Warfare. DTIC AD-770 735, US Army Chemical Research and Development Laboratories, Army Chemical Center, MD, 1960.
2. Herriott RM, Price WH. The formation of bacterial viruses in bacteria rendered non-viable by mustard gas. J Gen Physiol 1948;32,1:63–68.
3. Berger NA, Sikorski GW, Kurohara KK. Association of poly (adenosine, diphosphoribose) synthesis with DNA damage and repair in human lymphocytes. J Clin Invest 1979;63,6:1164–1171.
4. Meier HL, Johnson JB. Inhibitors of poly (ADP-ribose) polymerase prevent the cytotoxic effects induced in human lymphocytes by the alkylating agent, 2,2'-dichlorodiethyl sulfide (sulfur mustard, HD). Toxicol Applied Pharm 1992;113,2:234–239.
5. Meier HL, Gross CL, Papirmeister B. 2,2'-Dichlorodiethyl sulfide (sulfur mustard) decreases NAD$^+$ levels in the human leukocytes. Toxicol Lett 1987;39,no. 1:109–122.

6. Meier HL, Clayson ET, Kelly SA, Corun CM. Effect of sulfur mustard (HD) on ATP levels of human lymphocytes cultured in vitro. In Vitro Toxicol Mol Cell Toxicol 1996;9,2:135–139.

7. Millard CB, Meier HL, Broomfield CA. Exposure of human lymphocytes to an alkylating agent solubilizes truncated histone H2B. Biochim Biophys Acta 1994;1224,3:389–394.

8. Tomei LD, Cope FO. Current Communications. In: Cell and Molecular Biology, vol. 8, Cold Spring Harbor Laboratory Press, Cold Spring Harbor, NY, 1994.

21 DNA Repair Enzymatic Response in Cultured Human Epidermal Keratinocytes Following Sulfur Mustard Exposure

K. Ramachandra Bhat, PHD,
Betty J. Benton, BS,
and Radharaman Ray, PHD

CONTENTS

INTRODUCTION
METHODS
RESULTS
DISCUSSION
REFERENCES

INTRODUCTION

Use of live animals in toxicity testing, such as in the Draize test, is common in the cosmetics industry. For the past few years, the need to develop alternatives to animal testing has been well recognized by academia and industry. The motivating forces have been a greater social awareness of animal welfare and the economics of animal use. The most plausible and obvious choice is cultured animal cells or amphibian embryos, which can offer measurable biological responses to the actions of irritants and toxicants.

METHODS

When cultured human cells are exposed to irritants and toxicants, the cell's metabolic activity may be affected. The cells may respond to an

From: *Toxicity Assessment Alternatives: Methods, Issues, Opportunities*
Edited by: H. Salem and S. A. Katz © Humana Press Inc., Totowa, NJ

Table 1
Decay Rate Constants for Activated DNA Ligase
in NHEK Under Different Experimental Conditions

Treatment	HD concentration, mM	Decay constant, h^{-1}[a]	Half-life, h
None	0.3	0.56 ± 0.05	1.24
None	1.0	0.51 ± 0.07	1.36
2 mM 3-AB	1.0	0.14 ± 0.03	4.95
50 μM BAPTA AM	1.0	0.18 ± 0.04	3.85

[a]$N = 3 \pm$ SEM.

insult or an injury either by activation or deactivation of the enzymes involved in the respective pathways to alleviate cell injury. Such model systems, therefore, may serve as alternatives to animal use to obtain a direct correlation between cause and effect. Of particular interest to this laboratory is the action of sulfur mustard (bis-[2-chloroethyl] sulfide, HD) on skin and other exposed parts of the body. The effects of HD on skin can be mimicked in the normal human epidermal keratinocyte (NHEK) culture model. HD is a vesicant and causes chromosomal DNA damage. It forms alkyl adducts with heterocyclic bases of DNA (1). As a consequence, it activates the DNA repair pathway. Following exposure of NHEK to HD, increases in DNA repair enzymes, poly(ADP-ribose) polymerase (PARP) (2) and DNA ligase (3), have been observed. Activation of DNA ligase and PARP has also been reported in human skin fibroblasts exposed to another alkylating agent, dimethyl sulfate (4,5). In the absence of repair of the damaged DNA, mutations and carcinogenesis may occur. To repair the DNA damage efficiently, both PARP and DNA ligase are required. The time-course of the enzymatic response to DNA damage is very rapid. DNA ligase is activated within 30 min or less. This rapid response may be exploited as a sensitive method to identify toxic cellular DNA-damaging agents using cultured cell systems.

RESULTS

The HD activation of DNA ligase in NHEK has been thoroughly investigated in this laboratory (6,7), and the results suggest that monitoring DNA ligase activity in cultured NHEK or other human cell systems following exposure to toxic chemicals may provide a sensitive method to detect mutagens and carcinogens. In Table 1, the rate constants for the decay of the activated DNA ligase under different conditions are given. These rate constants were obtained by measuring the excess enzyme activity over identically treated "mock" controls as a function of time and treating the decrease of the enzyme activity as a first-order decay. An examination of the decay constant of HD-activated DNA ligase shows a half-life of 1.4 h, which permits the measurement of the enzyme activation following DNA damage in a reasonable time frame after the exposure. The decay constant was lower in the presence of either the PARP inhibitor 3-AB or the intracellular calcium chelator 1,2 *bis*(2 amino phenoxy) methane N,N,N',N' tetraacetic acid, tetraacetoxy methyl ester (BAPTA AM). The lowering of the rate of deactivation suggests that the lifetime of the DNA repair pathway is prolonged. The prolonged DNA repair pathway may enhance the viability of the cells.

DISCUSSION

Significant changes in the decay constant may also be indicative of interference by components present in the test material, and may therefore be used to detect the presence of DNA ligase inhibitors or synergistically acting components in the test material.

REFERENCES

1. Papirmeister B, Feister AJ, Sabina IR, Ford RD. Chemistry of sulfur mustard. In: Medical Defense Against Mustard Gas. CRC, Boca Raton, FL, 1991, pp. 102–109.
2. Clark O, Smith WJ. Activation of poly(ADP-ribose) polymerase by sulfur mustard in Hela cell cultures. Proceedings of the 1993 Medical Defense Bioscience Review, USAMRICD, APG, MD, 1:199–205, ADA 275667, 1993.
3. Bhat KR, Ray R. Sulfur mustard (HD) causes DNA ligase activation in normal human epidermal keratinocytes (NHEK). FASEB J 1995;9(3):A425.
4. James MR, Lehmann AR. Role of (poly adenosine diphosphate ribose) in deoxyribonucleic acid repair in human fibroblasts. Biochemistry 1982;21:4007–4013.
5. Bhat R, Subbarao SC. Adenosine diphosphate ribose polymerase (ADPR polymerase) and DNA ligase are linked during human DNA Repair. Proc Am Assoc Cancer Res 1990;31:3.
6. Bhat KR, Benton BJ, Ray R. Studies on DNA ligase in human skin cells exposed to sulfur mustard. Proceedings of the 1996 Medical Defense Bioscience Review, USAMRICD, APG, MD, 1996;2:767–776, AD A321841.
7. Bhat KR, Benton BJ, Ray R. DNA ligase activation following sulfur mustard exposure in cultured human epidermal keratinocytes. In Vitro Mol Toxicol 1998; 11(1):45–53.

22 Human Hepatocytes
A Novel Animal Alternative

John C. Lipscomb, PhD
and Patricia D. Confer, BS

CONTENTS

INTRODUCTION
METHODS
RESULTS
DISCUSSION
ACKNOWLEDGMENTS
REFERENCES

INTRODUCTION

Present cries for the end of animal experimentation are becoming louder and reaching more influential ears. The number of animals used by Department of Defense (DoD) research has decreased in the past two years in an appreciable manner. The rapidity at which animal use can be continually decreased relies on the development and validation of alternatives. Some of the proposed alternatives make use of entirely new technology, at increased cost, while still not eliminating the uncertainty of extrapolation of results from the experimental model to the human.

In this chapter, we have reviewed and examined the ability of the human hepatocyte and microsomal preparations to catalyze the bioactivation of a common groundwater contaminant, trichloroethylene (TRI). This bioactivation is catalyzed by cytochrome P450 2E1 *(1,2)*, an enzyme embedded in the endoplasmic reticulum that is concentrated in the microsomal fraction of cellular homogenates. We have previously examined the ability of human hepatic microsomes to metabolize TRI

From: *Toxicity Assessment Alternatives: Methods, Issues, Opportunities*
Edited by: H. Salem and S. A. Katz © Humana Press Inc., Totowa, NJ

(3) and sought to evaluate this bioactivation in a more physiologically relevant system, the intact liver cell. The attractiveness of metabolism and toxicity studies with human hepatocytes is that there is no need for cross-species extrapolation of results. Because multiple pathways and events are possible with the combined contents of the cell, a more relevant representation of the intact liver is possible. Because human hepatocytes are now available from a variety of sources, their use in metabolism and toxicity studies should increase.

We have evaluated TRI's metabolism in two in vitro human liver preparations: the isolated hepatocyte and the microsomal suspension. A potential disadvantage of the isolated hepatocyte is that its removal from the surrounding liver matrix may be damaging to the cell. When a compound's mechanism of toxic action involves metabolic activation, results from damaged systems may result in falsely low predictions of toxicity. Correlation of metabolic rates among in vitro systems will foster confidence in resulting data.

The advent of physiologically based pharmacokinetic modeling (PBPK) and its acceptance by regulators has resulted in the application of this technique in risk assessments. One limitation of modeling the human is verification by conducting human exposures. This is not possible with intrinsically toxic compounds. Carefully controlled exposures of humans to TRI have been accomplished, and the resulting data are being used to construct PBPK models. Additional data sets on plasma distribution profiles of parent compound and metabolites in TRI-exposed humans will be used to validate the model. Recently, metabolism constants derived in vitro have been used in the construction of a PBPK model for perchloroethylene *(4)*. TRI and perchloroethylene offer a unique situation where the human can be ethically exposed, and data can be used to validate appropriate models. We have evaluated the metabolism of TRI in both human microsomes and hepatocytes, and have compared the results, based on microsomal protein content. These data support the conclusion that TRI is metabolized at similar rates in microsomes and hepatocytes and strengthen the value of metabolic data derived from these in vitro systems.

METHODS

Chemicals

All chemicals were at least reagent grade and were obtained from Sigma Chemical Co. (St. Louis, MO) or Aldrich Chemical Co. (Milwaukee, WI) unless otherwise noted. Glucose-6-phosphate and NADP$^+$ were obtained from Boehringer-Mannhein (Indianapolis, IN).

Table 1
Human Microsome Donor Information

Donor	Smoking habits	Drinking habits
47 C M[a]	1ppd[b]	Social[c]
60 C M	2.5 ppd	Occasional
25 C M	None	Yes
43 C M	None	Heavy
51 C M	None	Yes
24 H M	None	Social
43 H M	None	Previous
50 C F	None	None

[a]Age in years. Ethnic origin: C, Caucasian; H, Hispanic. Sex: M, male; F, female.
[b]Smoking habit is reported in packs/d (ppd)
[c]Drinking habit was reported by family members.

Microsome Preparation and TRI Exposures

Human microsomes obtained from a commercial supplier (International Institute for the Advancement of Medicine, Exton, PA) were prepared via the method of Guengerich (5). Donor information is presented in Table 1. Microsomes were prepared from the livers of adult male Fischer 344 rats and B6C3F1 mice under identical procedure. Microsomal protein content was determined by the BCA method with bovine serum albumin as a standard. Total P450 was determined using the differential spectrophotometric method of Omura and Sato (6). TRI was dissolved in acetone and 1.0-µL injections were made directly into a 1.0-mL suspension containing microsomes, an nicotine adenine dinucleotide phosphate, reduced (NADPH)-regenerating system glucose-6-phosphate [G-6-P], NADP+, and G-6-P dehydrogenase), and Tris buffer, pH 7.4. Incubations were accomplished in 12.5-mL serum vials crimp-sealed with Teflon-lined rubber septa, maintained under gentle shaking at 37°C. Chloral hydrate (CH) and trichloroethanol formed were extracted with the addition of 2 vol of ethyl acetate. Ethyl acetate was analyzed by gas chromatography as detailed below.

Human Hepatocytes and TRI Exposures

Hepatocytes were obtained from human liver donors, and prepared by collagenase perfusion and isolation (Human Cell Culture Center, Anatomic Gift Foundation, Folkston, GA). Donor information is presented in Table 2. Cells were suspended in transport medium and shipped same-day air to our laboratory. The time from organ removal to in vitro

Table 2
Human Hepatocyte Donor Information

Donor[a]	Cause of death[b]
50 C M	CHI/MVA
48 H F	ICH
62 C F	ANOXIA
34 H M	ANOXIA
19 C M	GSW-H
72 C M	ICH

[a]Age in years. Sex: M, male; F, female.
Ethnic origin: C, Caucasian; H, Hispanic.
[b]Cause of death: CHI, closed head injury;
MVA, motor vehicle accident; ICH, intracranial hemorrhage; GSW-H, gunshot wound
to the head.

experiment did not exceed 36 h. Hepatocytes were analyzed initially for viability by trypan blue exclusion and were discarded if viability index was below 70%. Cells were incubated at a density of 2×10^6/mL in Chee's modified medium in 30-mL screw-capped Erlenmeyer flasks under either room air or purged with 95% O_2/5% CO_2. TRI was volatilized into tedlar bags containing known volumes of air and diluted into the sealed flasks to yield headspace concentrations of 25–10,000 ppm. Incubations were carried out for up to 2 h, and the reaction quenched by boiling. Toxicity was evaluated by monitoring the release of aspartate amino transferase (AST), alanine amino transferase (ALT), and lactate dehydrogenase (LDH) into media.

Partitioning of TRI

Chee's modified medium (Gibco, Grand Island, NY) with and without heat-inactivated cells was exposed to TRI in headspace, and partition coefficient was calculated by the method of Sato and Nakajima *(7)*. This value was used to estimate the intracellular TRI concentration.

Analysis of P450-Derived Metabolites

Following heat inactivation of hepatocytes, samples were split for CH analysis and for trichloroacetic acid (TCA)/trichloroethanol (TCOH) analysis. For CH and free TCOH analysis (hepatocytes and microsomes), samples were extracted with ethyl acetate, and 1.0 µL of the ethyl acetate extract was analyzed. For total TCOH and TCA analysis, samples were acidified and extracted into hexane, and derivitized with dimethylsulfate following modifications of the published methods *(8)*.

Liquid analysis of hexane and ethyl acetate extracts was performed using a Hewlett-Packard Model 7673A liquid injector connected with a Hewlett-Packard (Avondale, PA) Model 5890 Series II gas chromatograph interfaced with an electron-capture detector. Signal was integrated by a PE Nelson integrator (P E Nelson, Cupertino, CA). Chromatographic separation was performed on a Vocol capillary column (0.53 mm × 30 m, Supelco, Bellefonte, PA). Samples were quantified against an external standard curve of authentic compounds.

Quantification of Microsomal Protein in Hepatocytes

Nine grams of human liver were homogenized and the volume determined. Aliquots of the crude homogenate were saved, and microsomes were prepared from the rest. Homogenate and microsomal protein contents were determined and G-6-P activity (an activity catalyzed exclusively by microsomal protein) was measured under a broad range of substrate concentrations in microsomes and homogenate. Microsomal and homogenate proteins were serially diluted, and 10-µL aliquots analyzed for G-6-P activity by incubating for 30 min at 37°C with 10 µL 125 mM cacodylic acid, 0.125 mM EDTA, pH 6.5, 10 µL 50 mM Tris-acetate, 20% glycerol, pH 7.4, 70 µL 42.3 mM G-6-P. The reaction was quenched and developed by the addition of 1.0 mL reagent containing 2.25 mM ammonium molybdate, 2.2% sodium dodecyl sulfate, and 1.1% ascorbic acid. A standard curve of serial dilutions of authentic phosphate (potassium phosphate) was prepared, and quenching reagent was added as above. Samples and standards were allowed to develop in the dark at room temperature for 6 h prior to analysis. Intensity of standards and product was measured at 820 nm in a Beckman DU-650 recording spectrophotometer. The quantity of microsomal protein present per gram intact tissue was accomplished by multiplying the total activity (nmol/min/mg protein) in liver homogenate by the quantity of total protein per gram tissue. This total G-6-P activity (µmol/min/g tissue) was divided by the specific G-6-P activity of microsomes (nmol/min/mg microsomal protein) to produce the quantity of microsomal protein/g liver tissue. Microsomal protein content (mg microsomal protein/gram tissue) was divided into the hepatocyte density (125×10^6 cells/gram liver), to estimate the concentration of microsomal protein/hepatocyte. The resulting microsomal protein content was used to compare TRI metabolic activity across the two preparations.

Statistical Evaluation

Student's t-test was performed using SigmaStat (Jandel Scientific, San Rafael, CA) on an IBM PC. Significance was determined at $p \le 0.05$).

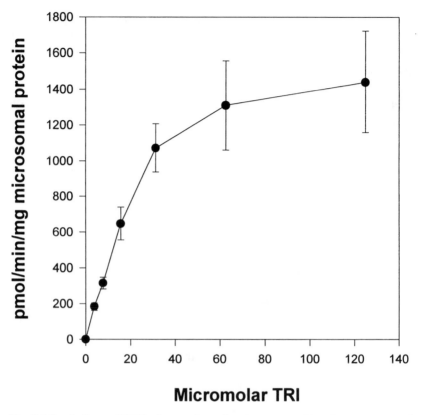

Micromolar TRI

Fig. 1. Metabolism of TRI by human hepatic microsomes. Results are presented as mean ± SD ($n = 8$) pmol TRI metabolized/min/mg microsomal protein. Data are consistent with reported K_m and V_{max} values for human microsomes.

RESULTS

The incubation of human hepatic microsomes ($n = 8$) indicated saturable TRI metabolism in this system (Fig. 1). We evaluated the metabolism of TRI in human hepatocytes ($n = 6$) under conditions that also attained intracellular concentrations greatly above the K_m value (25 μM) for humans *(3)*. The comparison of partition coefficients for TRI into media with and without cells was used to determine that the partition coefficient of TRI into hepatocytes was 21.62. This value was used to estimate the concentration of TRI in hepatocytes exposed to TRI in headspace:

$$[\{(5000 \text{ ppm} \times 5.35 \text{ mg TRI/m}^3/\text{ppm})/ \\ 1000 \text{ L/m}^3\}/131.4 \text{ mg/millimole}] \times 21.62 = 4.40 \text{ m}M \qquad (1)$$

An extraction of TRI from control medium and medium containing heat-inactivated hepatocytes confirmed this estimate.

The recovery of G-6-P activity in microsomes and crude homogenate in four liver samples indicates that 20.80 (±5.04 SD) mg microsomal protein are present/g of liver. Dividing 20.80 mg microsomal protein/g by 125×10^6 hepatocytes/g indicates that 0.166 mg microsomal protein is present in one million isolated hepatocytes. A comparison of the rates of metabolism in cells and prepared microsomes was based on quantification of microsomal protein. Data presented in Table 3 indicate that 2 million cells contain approx 0.333 mg microsomal protein. Metabolic rate (pmol/min/mg microsomal protein) obtained from microsomes under saturating concentrations (125 µM) of TRI was expressed as nmol/h/0.334 mg microsomal protein and compared again to the rate (nmol/h) seen in 2 million cells exposed to 5000 ppm TRI (4.40 mM intracellular concentration). Data presented in Fig. 2 indicate that the rates expressed in these two systems was not significantly different.

Data presented in Fig. 3 indicate that human hepatic microsomes metabolize significantly less TRI to CH than do either rat or mouse liver microsomes when exposed to TRI at fivefold above the K_m value.

DISCUSSION

The bioactivation of TRI involves an initial P450-mediated conversion to CH (1,2), which is then metabolized to TCA, TCOH, and dichloroacetic acid (DCA) (among others) (9,10). Some of these compounds have been demonstrated to produce toxic consequences associated with TRI exposure (11,12). The modulation of P450-dependent TRI metabolism in vivo (13) and in vitro (14) has been shown to modulate TRI's toxicity. We have shown that human hepatic microsomes metabolize much less TRI than microsomes from either the rat or mouse in vitro (15). These data may indicate that the human forms CH, TCA, TCOH, and DCA less efficiently than either the rat or mouse. Whether this effect is observed in the intact animal cannot be ascertained from these data alone, but hepatic metabolism in vivo is clearly reflected in hepatocyte incubations in vitro (16). Further, interspecies differences in predominant metabolic pathways are reflected in hepatocyte incubations (17). However, factors governing the distribution of TRI from the portal of entry to the liver may also be responsible for some species-related differences in vivo.

We have demonstrated a proportionate increase in metabolite formed in the presence of $0.5–2.0 \times 10^6$ cells/mL and from 0 to 2 h of incubation (not shown). We report a rate of 12.1-nmol product (CH, TCOH, and

Table 3
Estimation of Microsomal Protein in Hepatocytes

Human number	080195	100795	041895	072495	Mean	S.D.
Hepatic protein						
Sample mass (g)	9.385	9.473	9.173	9.012	9.261	0.208
Homogenate volume (mL)	40.0	38.9	38.0	35.0	38.0	2.15
Homogenate protein (mg/mL)	36.29	40.69	26.75	43.19	36.7	7.24
Protein recovery (mg/g)	154.7	167.1	110.8	167.7	150.1	26.9
G-6-P activity—liver homogenate						
nmol/min/mg protein	123	115	99.7	113	112.7	9.7
μmol/min/g liver	19.03	19.21	11.05	22.30	17.90	4.81
Microsomal protein						
Protein concentration (mg/mL)	11.76	12.21	5.38	10.35	9.25	3.13
G-6-P activity—microsomal protein						
(nmol/min/mg protein)	884	1034	706	812	859	138
Microsomal protein/g liver (mg/g)[a]	21.52	18.58	15.65	27.46	20.80	5.04
Million cells/g[b]					125×10^6	
Microsomal protein (mg MS protein/2.0×10^6 cells)[c]	0.344	0.297	0.250	0.439	0.333	0.081

[a]Determined by dividing total liver G-6-P activity (μmol/min/g liver) by microsomal G-6-P specific activity (nmol/min/mg microsomal protein).
[b]Hepatocyte density based on density of liver at 1 g/cm^3 and hepatocyte diameter of 13 μm.
[c]Determined by dividing mg microsomal protein/g by 125×10^6 hepatocytes/g.

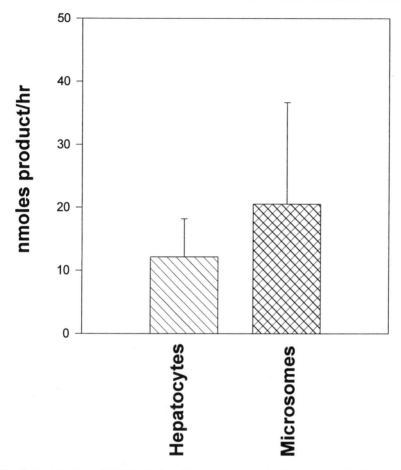

Fig. 2. Metabolism of TRI by isolated hepatocytes and microsomes of the human. Results are presented as mean ± SD (n = 8 microsomes and n = 6 hepatocytes) nmol product formed/h/0.333 mg microsomal protein and nmol product formed/h/2.0 × 10^6 isolated hepatocytes. Means were not significantly different (p = 0.256). Data indicate similar rates of metabolism in these two preparations.

TCA) formed/h from incubations containing 2 × 10^6 cells/mL. Our rates of TRI metabolism are confirmed by other reports of saturable TRI metabolism in human and rat hepatocytes *(18)*. These authors report a 11.3-nmol product formed from TRI metabolism in the human hepatocyte in 2 h from 1 × 10^6 cells. Agreement between the values reported for human hepatocyte TRI metabolism from these two studies and the lower rates of TRI metabolism in human compared to rat hepatocytes *(18)* and in human compared to rat and mouse microsomes *(15)* indicates that TRI biotransformation in human liver preparations does not

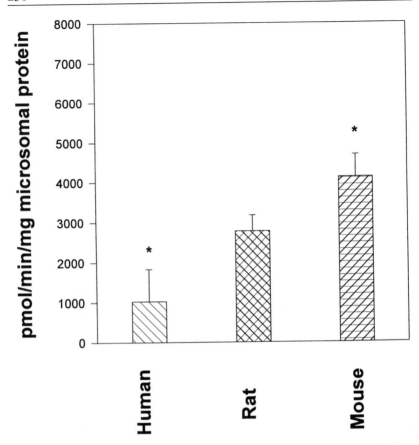

Fig. 3. Metabolism of TRI by rat, mouse, and human hepatic microsomes. Data are presented as nmol product formed/min/mg microsomal protein under saturating concentrations (125 μM TRI). Results demonstrate a lower rate of microsomal TRI metabolism in the human ($n = 8$) compared with the rat ($n = 3$ samples, each sample represented pooled microsomes from 3 rats) and mouse ($n = 3$ samples, each sample represented pooled microsomes from 5 mice). *Significantly different from rat, $p \leq 0.05$.

proceed at the rate observed in rodent liver preparations. The findings of Billings et al. *(16)* invite the extrapolation of these data to the intact organisms, with the resulting conclusion that humans are less well suited for TRI biotransformation than rodents.

Because we have quantified microsomal protein in the isolated hepatocyte, and evaluated TRI metabolism in both preparations under saturating conditions, we can compare metabolic rates on a "per-mg microsomal protein" basis. Our data indicate that TRI metabolic rates are not significantly different between the two systems. Although no significant differences were noted, we had hypothesized that the metabolic rate may be significantly influenced by lipid content of the two systems. The higher lipid content of the cell (compared to the microsomal preparation) may be predicted to sequester the highly lipophylic TRI, reducing the quantity of TRI available for metabolism. Statistical evaluation did not confirm that hypothesis, but separate experiments (not shown) did confirm that increasing the lipid content of microsomal incubations produced significant reduction of TRI metabolic rate.

Because TRI metabolism to CH and TCOH depends on the initial microsomal P-450-mediated oxidation of TRI to CH, our observation of similar rates of TRI metabolism (nmol product/h/mg microsomal protein) in these two systems indicates that our method of microsomal protein recovery is accurate. This method may be readily applied to other tissues to determine the content of P450/g tissue. These data may be used to predict the site-specific metabolism of TRI, and may influence the perceived importance of extrahepatic TRI metabolism. CH produced from TRI by the lung during an inhalation exposure may serve as a substrate for blood-derived TCOH and TCA production (19). Finally, the range of TRI metabolism by both systems is consistent with estimates of CYP2E1 variability in the population (20).

These data have demonstrated that comparable rates of cytochrome P-450-dependent TRI metabolism are expressed in microsomes and isolated cells prepared from the human. This indicates that once delivered to the liver, such factors as protein binding, competing enzyme pathways, or sequestration by lipids (as might have occurred in the isolated hepatocyte) may have a minimal effect on the P-450-dependent TRI metabolic pathway leading to TCOH, TCA, and DCA production. Our lack of demonstration of DCA in either human preparation is consistent with the lack of quantifiable concentrations of DCA in plasma of humans exposed to TRI. These factors may indicate that TRI metabolism studies conducted in microsomal preparations provide physiologically relevant data. Because we have previously demonstrated a K_m value of 20–60 μM TRI in 23 human microsomal samples (3), this value may govern TRI metabolism in vivo. The extrapolation of V_{max} data based on recovery of microsomal protein may provide data (mg metabolized/h/kg body wt) for direct input into PBPK models for TRI, as has been accomplished with perchloroethylene (4). Modeling of metabolic parameters can be accomplished through the application of Monte Carlo simulation to the variation of TRI metabolic parameters demonstrated in a sample of human hepatic microsomes (3), as has recently been accomplished in the physiologically based model developed for toluene (21).

The validation of such in vitro systems as these will promote their acceptance. When systems such as these become widely available and increase in use and acceptance, the application of data derived from them will reduce the costs and risks associated with experiments involving human exposure and the uncertainty produced by the extrapolation of rodent data. It is clear that many types of data can be gained from carefully constructed in vitro experiments. Further efforts to validate the application of human hepatocytes to toxicity and chemical metabolism will aid the acceptance of in vitro techniques, such as the human hepatocyte.

ACKNOWLEDGMENTS

We appreciate the encouragement and guidance of Jeff Fisher, Richat Abbas, and John Frazier. We gratefully acknowledge the contributions of the analytical chemistry unit of the Toxicology Division, specifically Gerry Buttler, for chemical analysis. All animals used in this study were handled in accordance with the principles stated in the Guide for the Care and Use of Laboratory Animals, prepared by the Committee on Care and Use of Laboratory Animal Resources, National Research Council, DHHS, National Institute of Health Publication 86-23, 1985, and the Animal Welfare Act of 1966, as amended. We are sincerely grateful for the unselfish donation of human tissue and realize that without conscientious citizenry, projects like this are not possible. This project was funded by a grant from the Strategic Environmental Research and Development Fund (SERDP).

NOTE ADDED IN PROOF

We have continued this study and have estimated microsomal protein recoveries and hepatocyte density values in intact human liver based solely on results obtained from microsome and hepatocyte preparations derived from four matching human liver samples. The distribution of microsomal protein to hepatocytes was determined to be 0.179 mg microsomal protein per million hepatocytes. When this value was used to compare metabolic rates (V_{max} values) observed in microsomes and expressed per unit microsomal protein with V_{max} values observed in hepatocytes and expressed per million cells, the values were remarkable similar (22). When metabolic rates (V_{max} values) were extrapolated from these in vitro preparations to the intact human, based on parameters used in corresponding PBPK models for the human (23), we found that our V_{max} values extrapolated to approximately 6.9 mg/hkg (22) and agreed closely with the modeled value (approximately 14 mg/hkg).

Finally, a better controlled set of human exposures to TRI has now been conducted and the results used to construct a more refined PBPK model for the human (24), in which the authors estimate V_{max} near 4–5 mg/hkg. These results demonstrate the usefulness of in vitro metabolic studies in the prediction of in vivo metabolic capacity.

REFERENCES

1. Guengerich FP, Kim DH, Iwasaki M. Role of human cytochrome P-450 IIE1 in the oxidation of many low molecular weight cancer suspects. Chem Res Toxicol 1991;4:168–179.
2. Leibman KH. Metabolism of trichloroethylene in liver microsomes. II. Identification of the reaction product as chloral hydrate. Mol Pharmacol 1965;1:239–246.
3. Lipscomb JC, Garrett CM, Snawder JE. Cytochrome P450 dependent metabolism of trichloroethylene: Interindividual differences in humans. Toxicol Appl Pharmacol 1997;142:311–318.
4. Reitz RH, Gargas ML, Mendrala AL, Schumann AM. In vivo and in vitro studies of perchloroethylene metabolism for physiologically based pharmacokinetic modeling in rats, mice and humans. Toxicol Appl Pharmacol 1996;136:289–306.
5. Guengerich FP. Analysis and characterization of enzymes. In: Hayes AW, ed. Principles and Methods of Toxicology, 2nd ed. Raven, New York, 1989, pp. 777–814.
6. Omura T, Sato R. The carbon monoxide binding pigment of liver microsomes. I. Evidence for its hemoprotein nature. J Biol Chem 1964;239:2370–2378.
7. Sato A, Nakajima T. A vial-equilibration method to evaluate the drug-metabolizing enzyme activity for volatile hydrocarbons. Toxicol Appl Pharmacol 1979;47:41–46.
8. Maiorino RM, Gandolfi AJ, Sipes IG. Gas chromatographic method for the halothane metabolites, trifluoroacetic acid and bromide, in biological fluids. Anal Toxicol 1980;4:250–254.
9. Sellers EM, Lang-Sellers M, Koch-Weser J. Comparative metabolism of chloral hydrate and trichlorofos. J Clin Pharmacol 1978;18:457–461.
10. Abbas RR, Seckel CS, Kidney JK, Fisher JW. Pharmacokinetic analysis of chloral hydrate and its metabolism in B6C3F1 mice. Drug Metab Dispos, 1996;24:1340–1346.
11. Daniel FB, DeAngelo AB, Stober JA, Olson GR, Page NR. Hepatocarcinogenicity of chloral hydrate, 2-chloroacetaldehyde, and dichloroacetic acid in the male B6C3F1 mouse. Fundam Appl Toxicol 1992;19:159–168.
12. DeAngelo AB, Daniel FB, Stober JA, Olson GR. The carcinogenicity of dichloroacetic acid in the male B6C3F1 mouse. Fundam Appl Tox 1991;16:337–347.
13. Buben JA, O'Flaherty EJ. Delineation of the role of metabolism in the hepatotoxicity of trichloroethylene and perchloroethylene: a dose–effect study. Toxicol Appl Pharmacol 1985;78:105–122.
14. Klaunig JE, Ruch RJ, Lin EC. Effects of trichloroethylene and its metabolites on rodent hepatocyte intercellular communication. Toxicol Appl Pharmacol 1989;99: 454–465.
15. Lipscomb JC, Garrett CM, Snawder JE. Use of kinetic and mechanistic data in species extrapolation of bioactivation: cytochrome P-450 dependent krichloroethylene metabolism at occupatlionally releuant concentrations. J Occup Health 1998;40:110–117.

16. Billings RE, McMahon RE, Ashmore J, Wagle SR. The metabolism of drugs in isolated hepatocytes: A comparison with *in vivo* drug metabolism and drug metabolism in subcellular fractions. Drug Metab Dispos 1977;5:518–526.

17. Green CE, LeValley S, Tyson CA. Comparison of amphetamine metabolism using isolated hepatocytes from five species including human. J Pharmacol Exp Ther 1986;237:931–936.

18. Knadle SA, Green CE, Baugh M, Vidensek M, Short SM, Partos X, et al. Trichloroethylene biotransformation in human and rat primary hepatocytes. Toxicol In Vitro 1990;4:537–541.

19. Lipscomb JC, Mahle DA, Brashear WT, Garrett CM. A species comparison of chloral hydrate metabolism in blood and liver. Biochem Biophys Res Commun 1996;227:340–350.

20. Barton HA, Flemming CD, Lipscomb JC. Evaluating human variability in chemical risk assessment: hazard identification and dose-response assessment for noncancer oral toxicity of trichloroethylene. Toxicology 1996;110:271–287.

21. Pierce CH, Dills RL, Morgan MS, Northstein GL, Shen DD, Kalman DA. Interindividual differences in 3H-toluene toxicokinetics assessed by a semiempirical physiologically based model. Toxicol Appl Pharmacol 1996;139:49–61.

22. Lipscomb JC, Fisher JW, Confer PD, Byczkowski JZ. In vitro to in vivo extrapolation for trichloroethylene metabolism in humans. Toxicol Appl Pharmacol 1998;152:376–387.

23. Allen B, Fisher JW. Pharmacokinetic modeling of trichloroethylene and trichloroacetic acid in humans. Risk Anal 1993;13:71–85.

24. Fisher JW, Mahle D, Abbas R. A human physiologically based pharmacokinetic model for trichloroethylene and its metabolites, trichloroacetic acid and free trichloroethanol. Toxicol Appl Pharmacol 1998;152:339–359.

V VALIDATION, REGULATORY ACCEPTANCE, AND ANIMAL PROTECTION PERSPECTIVES

23 An Animal Protection Perspective

Martin L. Stephens, PHD

CONTENTS

INTRODUCTION
THE HUMANE SOCIETY OF THE UNITED STATES (HSUS)
AND THE THREE Rs
GENERAL COMMENTS ON PROGRESS
SPECIFIC COMMENTS
CONCLUSIONS

INTRODUCTION

It should be emphasized at the outset that this chapter provides *an* animal protection perspective, and not *the* animal protection perspective. Animal protection organizations differ in their commitment to the Three R's approach, in terms of both their policies and their day-to-day activities. At one end of the spectrum, some organizations oppose the Three R's approach as a diversion from what they see as the primary issues; namely, the ethics and utility of animal research. At the other end, some organizations fully embrace the alternatives approach and devote virtually all of their day-to-day efforts to promoting this cause.

THE HUMANE SOCIETY OF THE UNITED STATES (HSUS) AND THE THREE RS

The Humane Society of the United States (HSUS) falls between these two ends of the spectrum. Although our work on animal research issues is not limited to promoting the Three Rs, the alternatives approach is a key component of our policy and activity on these issues. In our view, the alternative approach provides an important part of the framework for reducing the suffering and killing of animals in laboratories.

From: *Toxicity Assessment Alternatives: Methods, Issues, Opportunities*
Edited by: H. Salem and S. A. Katz © Humana Press Inc., Totowa, NJ

The HSUS has been at the forefront of the animal protection community's efforts to promote alternative methods. It bestows the Russell and Burch Award annually to scientists who have made outstanding contributions to the Three Rs. It has partnerships with the Gillette Corporation as well as key institutional players on the alternatives scene, including the Interagency Coordinating Committee for the Validation of Alternative Methods (ICCVAM), the Interagency Regulatory Alternatives Group (IRAG), the Center for Alternatives to Animal Testing (CAAT), and the European Centre for the Validation of Alternative Methods (ECVAM). Also, it has been a part of the Army's biennial conferences on alternatives for the past several years.

GENERAL COMMENTS ON PROGRESS

First, some general remarks on what has been achieved to date in implementing the vision that William Russell and Rex Burch outlined in their landmark book of 1959, *The Principles of Humane Experimental Technique*. The HSUS is heartened by several positive developments, including the following:

- The increasing number of scientists and corporations that are developing and implementing alternative methods, or funding such work.
- The institutionalization of alternatives methods through the creation of such centers as CAAT, ICCVAM, and ECVAM.
- The undertaking of major validation studies and efforts to harmonize national guidelines on validation and regulatory acceptance.

On the other hand, the alternatives community has little to show for its efforts in the way of validated and accepted replacement alternatives. Until it does, it is not likely to win over those skeptical or indifferent to the alternatives approach in the animal protection community and among the general public.

Perhaps too much reliance is being placed on animal data as the standard against which to judge the performance of potential replacements. Based on Leon Bruner's analyses, animal data on eye irritation appear to be too variable even to allow for the possibility of a good correlation between in vivo and in vitro results.

These general remarks serve as the backdrop for specific comments on efforts in alternatives.

SPECIFIC COMMENTS

One of the IRAG's assessment of eye irritation alternatives findings is the realization that industry has been making fairly widespread use of in vitro methods, although as screens, and not as replacements.

On the downside, some observers, the author included, have felt uncomfortable with the IRAG's heavy emphasis on numerical Draize scores. Given the considerable variability of Draize results, these scores should not be taken too seriously. Some observers also had hoped that the IRAG evaluation would at least help in identifying suitable alternatives for detecting severe irritants. Unfortunately, the IRAG appears not to have addressed this important issue.

The results of the European Community/Home Office (ECHO) validation study of alternatives to the Draize test were discouraging. Although a great deal of money was spent, and some of the best minds had planned the study that was conducted in many good laboratories using the most promising alternative methods, we still do not have a validated alternative, or battery of alternatives to the Draize test.

However, we can take heart in the new level of sophistication that the ECHO study brought to the challenge of validation. Prevalidation studies led to a fine-tuning of the assays prior to the full-blown (and expensive) validation. The validation itself employed a prediction model to generate testable hypotheses and a framework for interpreting the data.

Despite its disappointing results, many American animal protectionists view the ECHO study as an example of a greater commitment to the alternatives approach on the part of the government in Europe, as compared to the US.

The European Cosmetic, Toiletry and Perfumery Association's (COLIPA) validation of eye irritation alternatives confirmed that industry is indeed employing in vitro methods as screens, as the IRAG study had found. Presumably, this practice is decreasing animal use. The COLIPA program also has some of the same sophisticated elements as the ECHO study, including a prediction model.

Many animal protectionists view the COLIPA study as a direct response to public pressure against animal testing in Europe, pressure that led to the European legislation against animal testing of cosmetics. Consequently, the study is seen as an example of how activism can speed progress on alternatives. Animal protectionists await the final outcome of this project.

An informative update on the work of the ICCVAM and on the Organization for Economic Cooperation and Development (OECD) workshop on harmonization of validation and acceptance criteria for alternative toxicological test methods indicates that the federal government, through ICCVAM, has become an active player on the alternatives scene. Official government participation is essential to our efforts. It is also encouraging to have the international community, through

OECD, working on harmonizing criteria for the validation and regulatory acceptance of alternatives.

The International Life Sciences Institute (ILSI) should be congratulated for tapping the expertise of research ophthalmologists in its work on eye irritation testing. Too much of the work on eye irritation alternatives has proceeded without input from this important group. Research ophthalmologists might be able to help gather new or pre-existing human data to use as a true gold standard against which to compare animal and in vitro methods. The paradigm needs to be shifted away from using animal data as a default standard, since industry sells its products to people, not rabbits.

CONCLUSIONS

The updates provided in the preceding chapters indicate that some important and encouraging signs of progress are being made. Nonetheless, there are no dramatic announcements about any animal procedure being replaced by an innovative new alternative. In some ways, we are spinning our wheels, stuck at our current plateau of progress.

We in the alternatives community should acknowledge our limitations. We have limited resources. The alternatives approach, relatively speaking, has few adherents in academia, government, and even industry. We have few successes to point to, at least as reflected in the number of animal procedures completely replaced by nonanimal methods thanks to our efforts.

Given this situation, it is recommended that we focus our efforts on a small number of manageable goals. If we do not have the wherewithal to replace the Draize eye test completely soon, for example, then let us set interim goals, such as replacing this test for assessing severe irritants. If we are unlikely to hit home runs, let us stop trying to reach for the bleachers, and instead, try at least to hit some singles, doubles, and triples.

In the absence of dramatic announcements about progress, companies, national governments, and perhaps other stakeholders should publicize whatever gains are being made and lay out their plans for the future.

Despite these worries, the author remains optimistic about the future. The author is encouraged by the emerging partnerships among government, industry, academia, and animal protection. The alternatives approach, slowly but surely, is becoming mainstream. Progress is inevitable, but let us ensure that its pace is swift!

24 Federal Interagency Activities Toward Validation and Regulatory Acceptance of Alternative Tests

Errol Zeiger, PhD, JD

INTRODUCTION

During the past few years, there has been a tremendous amount of coordinated activity within the federal government regarding validation and regulatory acceptance of alternative testing methods. Much of this effort in test method validation and regulatory acceptance was initiated in response to a mandate to the National Institute of Environmental Health Sciences (NIEHS) in the 1993 National Institutes of Health (NIH) Revitalization Act (Table 1). In response to Section (b)(4) of this Act, an ad hoc Interagency Coordinating Committee on the Validation of Alternative Methods (ICCVAM) was established. It was made up of representatives of 15 federal research and regulatory agencies and organizations (ATSDR, CPSC, DoD, DoE, DoI, DoT, EPA, FDA, NCI, NIEHS, NIH, NIOSH, NLM, OSHA, and USDA), and chaired by Richard Hill, EPA and William Stokes, NIEHS.)

From: *Toxicity Assessment Alternatives: Methods, Issues, Opportunities*
Edited by: H. Salem and S. A. Katz © Humana Press Inc., Totowa, NJ

Table 1
The NIH Revitalization Act of 1993 Title XIII—
The National Institute of Environmental Health Sciences

"Sec. 463A. (a) There is established within the Institute a program for conducting applied research and testing regarding toxicology, which program shall be known as the Applied Toxicological Research and Testing Program.

"(b) In carrying out the program established under subsection (a), the Director of the Institute shall, with respect to toxicology, carry out activities—

1. to expand knowledge of health effects of environmental agents;
2. to broaden the spectrum of toxicology information that is obtained on selected chemicals;
3. to develop and validate assays and protocols, including alternative methods that can reduce or eliminate the use of animals in acute or chronic safety testing;
4. to establish criteria for the validation and regulatory acceptance of alternative testing and to recommend a process through which scientifically validated alternative methods can be accepted for regulatory use;
5. to communicate the results of research to government agencies, to medical, scientific, and regulatory communities, and to the public; and
6. to integrate related activities of the [DHHS]."

The goals of ICCVAM were to communicate federal government criteria and processes for review of toxicological test methods; encourage development of testing methods for improved risk assessment; provide guidance for scientists and regulatory agencies; increase regulatory acceptance of validated new methods; promote national and international harmonization; encourage refinement, reduction, and replacement of animal use; and encourage the use of validated and accepted methods.

The product of this interagency committee was a report that was endorsed by all the participating agencies, and sets forth guiding principles for scientific validation and regulatory acceptance. The report is designed to emphasize principles of validation and acceptance, be applicable to all toxicological testing methods, and be sufficiently flexible to meet future needs. An important consideration in the development of the report was that there were no existing formal agency criteria for judging the scientific validation of a new or revised test.

A National Toxicology Program (NTP) Workshop on the Validation and Regulatory Acceptance of Alternative Toxicological Testing Methods was held in December 1995, in Arlington, VA. Its purpose was to provide comments and recommendations on the ICCVAM draft report *(1)* from invited experts and the public. The workshop report was used in the preparation of the final ICCVAM report *(2)*.

The level of international activity in this area has also increased. At the time the ICCVAM report was being revised, the Organization for Economic Cooperation and Development (OECD) Workshop on Harmonization of Validation and Acceptance Criteria for Alternative Test Methods met in January 1996, in Solna, Sweden. Its purpose was to reach consensus on harmonized principles and criteria for validation and acceptance of toxicological test methods, with emphasis on alternative tests; to develop guidance for validation procedures; and to discuss general principles concerning strategies and schemes for risk assessment. The US is a member of the OECD and was a participant in the workshop.

This chapter describes the validation and regulatory acceptance criteria and processes recommended by the ICCVAM, discusses planned future activities in this area, and summarizes the efforts of the OECD to develop a document on validation and acceptance criteria for alternative methods.

ICCVAM COMMITTEE REPORT

Alternative test methods, as discussed in the Act, refer to tests that refine animal use (i.e., eliminate pain or discomfort), reduce animal use, or replace animals with nonanimal test systems or with animals lower on the phylogenetic scale. Because the requirements for scientific validity of alternative tests are no different that those required for any other type of toxicological tests, a decision was made to address toxicological tests in general, and not only those that met the criteria for alternatives.

The ICCVAM divided the processes into those that addressed the scientific validation of a new or revised method, and those involved in the regulatory acceptance of the method.

Validation is defined as the scientific process by which the reliability and relevance of a test method are established for a specific purpose. This process is universal; that is, standard guidelines can be developed for evaluating the operational parameters of a test procedure regardless of the use to which it will be put. The scientific validation procedures provide information on the reproducibility of the test, and how well it performs in identifying the chemicals or biological effects of interest. A test will not be tagged as "valid" or "not valid." Instead, its operational parameters will be characterized and made available to the individuals making the regulatory decisions. In a separate process, the regulatory agencies would then decide, with regard to the specific mandate of that agency, whether that test is adequate to support decisions regarding human or environmental exposure and risk.

(Regulatory) acceptance is defined as the process whereby a given test is considered suitable for risk-assessment purposes for the protection of human health or the environment. Validation is a prerequisite for regulatory acceptance. Regulatory acceptance criteria are, of necessity, less standard than validation criteria. Each regulatory agency operates under its own legislative mandates; in some cases, there are multiple laws governing the operation and regulatory authorities of a single agency. Each agency has its own concerns and needs, and regulatory requirements are different for different types of substances. For example, much more assurance of safety is needed for a substance that is going to be deliberately added to foods than for a substance that is only going to be handled by a few trained people under controlled conditions.

ICCVAM formed subcommittees to prepare the sections of the document that addressed Validation of Test Methods and Regulatory Acceptance of Toxicological Test Methods. Following the workshop that was held to provide public comment on the draft report, a third subcommittee was formed to prepare a report section on Future Directions and Implementation *(1)*.

Test Method Validation

The criteria for validation of new or revised test methods are summarized in Table 2. New tests can replace or be interchangeable with currently accepted methods, or can incorporate new end points that have no correlate in existing tests. The validation information required for a test will vary with the type and proposed use of the test. Three general types of tests could be considered for validation: definitive tests, screening tests, and adjunct tests.

Definitive tests provide data that are used to identify hazardous substances and to provide information that can be used in risk assessments. Screening tests are used for preliminary identification of potential adverse effects, or for selecting chemicals or setting priorities for definitive tests. They often provide only a qualitative or semiquantitative response. Adjunct tests are used to aid in the interpretation of results from other tests, or provide information related to the mechanism of toxicity, or relevance to humans.

The criteria for validation of a test are a function of the purpose for which it will be used. Tests where the mechanism of action is understood are generally easier to validate because their relevance to the biological effect of concern is easier to establish.

Table 2
ICCVAM Summary Criteria for Test Method Validation

Scientific and regulatory rationale
Biological basis/relationship to toxic effect of interest
Formal detailed protocol
Reliability assessed (intra- and interlaboratory reproducibility)
Relevance assessed (performance with appropriate reference chemicals)
Limitations identified
Data quality (ideally performed under Good Laboratory Practices [GLPs] regulations)
All data available for review
Independent scientific peer review

The components of a test validation procedure include a determination and measurement of intra- and interlaboratory reproducibility. The substances used for the validation procedure should be representative of the substances for which the test is designed. Attempts should be made to identify the chemical classes that cannot be adequately evaluated by the method. Where possible, the baseline reference for a new test should be the response of the species of interest. All data supporting claims about a new method must be available.

The test validation process should be highly flexible and adapted to the specific test method and proposed use. Despite the need for flexibility, the various components of the validation process must be included or addressed. Because tests can be used for different purposes by different types of organizations, and with varying categories of substances, the determination of whether a procedure is considered to be scientifically validated must be made on a case-by-case basis, in the context of the proposed use(s) of the test.

Regulatory Acceptance

The various US regulatory agencies have their responsibilities defined by legislative mandate, and their approaches to hazard and risk assessment are bound by those mandates, and the types and uses of substances that they regulate. As a result, they have different requirements for test data. A test may be accepted for some, but not all classes of chemicals or product lines. This section of the report describes the various criteria taken into consideration by regulatory agencies in their assessment of the utility of a proposed new test for hazard or risk assessment.

All test submissions for regulatory acceptance should identify the specific purpose the test serves in the overall risk-assessment process. The results of validation studies should be part of the submission package.

Table 3
ICCVAM Summary Criteria for Test Method Acceptance

Adequately predicts the toxic end point of interest
Generates data for risk-assessment purposes that
    Are at least as useful as data from existing methods/strategies;
    Provide a comparable or better level of protection of human health or the
    environment
There are adequate data for substances of interest to a regulatory program
Robust and transferable
Cost-effective and likely to be used
Refinement, reduction, and replacement of animal use considered

The acceptance criteria will depend on the type of test being proposed (adjunct vs definitive; mechanistic vs correlative) or the extent of modification being proposed for an existing test. A definitive test would require a higher level of validation than an adjunct test, particularly if it is proposed as a replacement for a traditional test. Data generated or reported according to Good Laboratory Practices (GLP) procedures carries a higher level of assurance. The criteria for regulatory acceptance are summarized in Table 3.

The committee made the following recommendations regarding the regulatory acceptance process:

Acceptance of new tests will be facilitated by a coordinated process of involvement and communication between all stakeholders at all stages of test development and validation.

A federal interagency committee should be established to coordinate exchange of information, test method validation, and related activities.

Agencies should develop internal, central clearing systems for evaluation of new and revised tests.

Test guidelines should be harmonized among agencies and among international organizations, as appropriate.

Future Directions and Implementation

It was recommended that there should be a standing, permanent, federal interagency coordinating committee through NIEHS/NTP. This committee would serve as an interagency clearinghouse to coordinate review of new methods and their data submissions with appropriate agencies. It would also serve as a communication link to government and nongovernment stakeholders at all stages of the development, validation, review, and acceptance process; facilitate communication and information sharing across government agencies and with outside stake-

Table 4
The OECD Steps in the Validation
and Acceptance of New Test Methods

Need identified
Research
Development
Prevalidation/test optimization
Validation
Review
Regulatory submission
Regulatory acceptance
Implementation

holders; coordinate technical reviews of proposed new and revised test methods; provide administrative guidance for validation and regulatory acceptance; foster interagency and international test method harmonization; develop guidance on related issues; and promote awareness of accepted methods.

This interagency committee would advance the overall goal of the ICCVAM effort, which is to facilitate validation and regulatory acceptance of new test methods that will provide for improved protection of human health and the environment, and improved animal welfare: refinement, reduction, and replacement.

OECD WORKSHOP ON HARMONIZATION OF VALIDATION AND ACCEPTANCE CRITERIA FOR ALTERNATIVE TOXICOLOGICAL TEST METHODS

The purpose of the workshop was to develop harmonized principles and criteria for validation and acceptance of new or revised testing methods. There were three breakout groups. They addressed Principles and Criteria for Validation and Acceptance, Practical Approaches to Validation, and Testing Strategies. The Workshop Report *(3)* will serve as the basis for a future OECD Guidance Document. The stages in the test validation process are summarized in Table 4.

Summary of OECD Working Group 1: Principles and Criteria for the Validation and Acceptance of New or Modified Toxicological Tests

The levels of assurance needed that a test is valid and appropriate will vary with its proposed uses. The decision criteria need to be flexible.

Adequate test data should be presented for substances representative of those administered by the regulatory program or agency. A clear statement of scientific need and regulatory purpose of the test must be available, and the relationship of the test end point to the biological effect of interest must be addressed. The performance of the method should have been evaluated in relation to existing toxicity data and information from the relevant target species. The test variability and reproducibility should be known, and its performance demonstrated using coded reference chemicals. The test must be robust and transferable, and allow for standardization. All data supporting the use of the test method must be available for review and should have been obtained in accordance with GLP principles.

Regulatory acceptance of a test is dependent on the outcome of scientific validation. The proposed test should provide data that predict the end point of interest, and demonstrate a link between the new and existing tests, or effects in the target species. For a new test to be accepted, there should be evidence that it provides data for risk assessment that give a comparable or better level of protection for human health or the environment than existing tests.

Summary of OECD Working Group 2:
Practical Approaches to Validation

The validation process is designed to establish the reliability and relevance of a method for a specifically defined purpose. It is not designed to develop or optimize protocols, but is a confirmation process designed to determine the operational parameters of the test and to define its usefulness.

There are three stages in the validation of a new test: the test development phase; the test optimization/prevalidation phase; and the validation phase. It is important that a method and its role in toxicological testing be well defined before being subjected to a formal validation. Many of these factors are addressed during the "test optimization" (prevalidation) phase. A management/planning team should oversee the formal validation phase, and a biostatistician should be an integral member of the process for the design of the study and the evaluation of the results.

Topics addressed in the report include: test definition; test optimization; assessment of readiness of the method for validation; planning the validation study; conduct of testing; statistical recommendations; and reporting of validation study results. Emphasis was placed on the need for peer review of the test protocol and data, and of the appropriateness of the prediction model used.

Summary of OECD Working Group 3:
Testing Strategies/Schemes to Be Applied for the Testing and Assessment of Chemicals and Chemical Products

Testing strategies should maximize use of existing knowledge; minimize use and suffering of animals; optimize use of resources; achieve appropriate and relevant risk assessments; and ensure that the data are internally consistent and mutually supportive. Preliminary testing strategies for eye irritation/corrosion and skin irritation/corrosion were developed.

The sequence of tests in a testing strategy should permit the prediction of adverse effects. They should also provide dose–response information to support quantitative risk assessment. Structure–activity relationships, data and knowledge bases, and existing test data should be used wherever possible. Where possible, testing strategies should incorporate tests of known and relevant mechanisms of action, and consideration should be given to multiple uses of data. Less stressful procedures and those using fewer animals, and validated alternatives to animals should be given preference.

Preference should be given to the components of a strategy that relate specifically to measures in humans, including the use of human tissue for in vitro tests. Where possible, the use of humans should be encouraged at an appropriate point in a strategy.

SUMMARY

The validation of a test method does not confer on that method a presumption that it is valid for all test chemicals and for all uses of the test data. The determination of the operating characteristics of a test allows the potential user of information from that test to determine whether the test meets the particular needs of the organization, or what situations are appropriate for the use of the test. The decision to use or not to use a particular test is highly subjective, and cannot be tied to a "checklist" of test attributes. To a great extent, acceptance of a test is a function of the level of comfort a regulator or a manager has with the information provided by the test, irrespective of its specific reproducibility or correlation frequencies.

The ICCVAM and OECD documents provide a basis and guidelines for the establishment of processes for the review and evaluation of new and revised test methods that are consistent among regulatory agencies, have lead to the establishment in the US of an interagency group to coordinate the evaluations of new tests. This will ease the burden on test developers, because they can now communicate with a single entity, rather than preparing submissions to each agency or program that might have use for the test. The formation of this interagency committee will ensure that each agency or program will not have to perform its own independent reviews on a newly submitted test, and will minimize the possibility of sending mixed signals to the test's developers and users.

The reports developed by the ICCVAM and the OECD will provide significant support to test developers. They will go a long way toward ensuring that the different regulatory organizations in the US and other countries will look at the same types of information when assessing the regulatory acceptability of the test results, and eliminating redundancy in test validation programs and in test submissions to agencies.

REFERENCES

1. Final Report: NTP Workshop on Validation and Regulatory Acceptance of Alternative Toxicological Test Methods. December 11–12, 1995, Arlington, VA. National Institute of Environmental Health Sciences, Research Triangle Park, NC, March 18, 1996.
2. Interagency Coordinating Committee on the Validation of Alternative Methods (ICCVAM), Validation and Regulatory Acceptance of Toxicological Test Methods. A report of the ad hoc Interagency Coordinating Committee on the Validation of Alternative Methods, National Institute of Environmental Health Sciences, NIH, DHHS, 1997. [Available on the internet at htt://ntp-server.niehs.nih.gov/htdocs/ICCVAM/ICCVAM.html]
3. Organization for International Cooperation and Development (OECD), Report of the OECD Workshop on harmonization of validation and acceptance criteria for alternative toxicological test methods. January 22–24 1996, Solna, Sweden. OECD, Paris, France, 1996.

INDEX